Practice Under Pressure

Critical Issues in Health and Medicine

Edited by Rima D. Apple, University of Wisconsin–Madison,
and Janet Golden, Rutgers University, Camden

Growing criticism of the U.S. healthcare system is coming from consumers, politicians, the media, activists, and healthcare professionals. Critical Issues in Health and Medicine is a collection of books that explores these contemporary dilemmas from a variety of perspectives, among them political, legal, historical, sociological, and comparative, and with attention to crucial dimensions such as race, gender, ethnicity, sexuality, and culture.

For a list of titles in the series, see the last page of the book.

Practice Under Pressure

Primary Care Physicians and Their Medicine in the Twenty-first Century

Timothy Hoff

Rutgers University Press

New Brunswick, New Jersey, and London

Library of Congress Cataloging-in-Publication Data

Hoff, Timothy, 1965–
   Practice under pressure : primary care physicians and their medicine in the twenty-first
century / Timothy Hoff.
      p. ; cm.—(Critical issues in health and medicine)
   Includes bibliographical references and index.
   ISBN 978-0-8135-4675-9 (hardcover : alk. paper) —
   ISBN 978-0-8135-4676-6 (pbk. : alk. paper)
   1. Primary care (Medicine)—United States. I. Title. II. Series: Critical issues in health
and medicine.
   [DNLM: 1. Primary Health Care—trends—United States.   2. Health Care Reform—United
States.   3. Physicians, Family—trends—United States. W 84.6 H698p 2010]
   RA427.9.H64 2010
   362.1—dc22   2009006058

A British Cataloging-in-Publication record for this book is available from the British Library.

Copyright © 2010 by Timothy Hoff

Visit our Web site: http://rutgerspress.rutgers.edu

Manufactured in the United States of America

For Sharon and Kieran

Contents

Preface

Why a book on primary care? Because there is no other part of the health care system that is in greater trouble right now, and no other part that plays such an important role in people's lives. Primary care always receives less attention than sexier specialty counterparts such as surgery and emergency medicine. A surgeon I once interviewed said his job consisted of "assaulting people." He said the hardest decision he had to make was in knowing when to assault patients for their own good and when to leave them alone. Now that sounds like an exciting, rewarding, difficult, and life-altering job for the person brave enough to do it.

I once observed a group of emergency room physicians do their work at a local academic medical center. In between the routine emergencies came patients with dramatic penetrating wounds from knives and gunshots, blunt traumas from car accidents and attempted suicides, and emergent abdominal pains just hours away from a burst appendix or acute pancreatitis. This work, while boring and frustrating at times, also sounds pretty stimulating given its unpredictability and time-sensitive nature. And because of this appeal, these types of medical specialties get a lot of attention in the press, on television, and by writers and academic researchers.

But primary care medicine is still the unsung hero of our health care system, and primary care physicians (PCPs) are its main caretaker. It is a field of medicine aimed at preventing us from getting sick and taking care of us in the early stages of illness to reduce the need for expensive and intrusive health care services. Too bad the notion of prevention is out of vogue in much of American society at present—a society that gets unhealthier by the year. Primary care physicians may not deal much with acute life-and-death situations, but they are more important than any other physician in giving us a chance to avoid serious procedures such as cardiac bypass surgery or the amputation of a limb due to diabetes complications.

The current medical scene is not a pretty picture for primary care physicians or the medicine they practice. It will not get significantly better in the near future. We talk about national health reform in this country, and about the theoretical importance of primary care in stemming runaway health inflation and enhancing people's lives. We talk about coming to the rescue with new money and gimmicky programs that are not based on any real evidence.

We introduce magic bullets like the medical home concept and electronic health records because they sound simple and appealing to everyone. But no one—politicians, the public, or the medical profession to name three key stakeholders—seems committed to doing what it takes to reposition generalist medicine at the center of U.S. health care delivery. No one seems willing to take the sustained action to move us away from high-tech, high-priced medical practice that keeps us waiting until we are sick or dying, and toward prevention-oriented medicine that requires us to take better care of ourselves while using primary care physicians as the experts who can help us do so.

Without such a collective will, we are left with the reality of today's inadequate primary care situation and are neglecting the incremental strategies that might help strengthen it. The following chapters tell the story, for better or worse, of how primary care work plays out in the early twenty-first century, and who the physicians are that currently do this work. I hope readers will conclude that as far as primary care is concerned, and health care generally, one must appreciate the deeper roots of the problem first, and know something about the people that must help solve that problem, before rushing to any solutions, big or small. There is no simple, quick fix to what ails primary care in the United States today. But if I were a surgeon and primary care medicine were my patient, I would venture that the time to assault it, for its own good, is now.

I am most grateful to the primary care physicians, medical students and residents, and medical leaders who gave of their time to be interviewed for this book. Their perspectives have taught me much about how health care can and should work. They are a busy group, and I feel lucky that I was able to speak with so many of them. I also wish to thank Doreen Valentine at Rutgers University Press who offered valuable feedback on the manuscript and pushed me to keep improving it. Most of all I want to thank my wife, Sharon, and son, Kieran, who kept my spirits up when the process of book writing got me down. They are an inspiration to me.

Timothy Hoff
Albany, New York
January 2009

Practice Under Pressure

Chapter 1

The Transformation of Primary Care in the United States

Primary care is undergoing profound change in the United States. This is evident in a sicker general population, a decreasing supply of doctors to care for that population, new alternatives to the traditional primary care physician and practice, and an economic model of primary care delivery that creates dissatisfied doctors and patients. Everyone from professional associations to the government believes that money is at the root of the problem. Primary care doctors get paid much less than other doctors, and primary care services are not valued in the same way by third-party payers as specialty services.

Money is only part of the problem. Focusing only on better reimbursement or salaries, as most solutions to the primary care crisis currently do, obscures the impact of an evolving primary care workforce, the negative effects of a reduced scope of work in primary care, and poorly designed primary care training that renders the field unattractive to aspiring doctors. Indeed, the field of primary care has contributed to its own continuing demise, handing over more sophisticated work like hospital medicine to others with little but a whimper. Primary care physicians play to financial incentives that produce eight-hour work days of seeing patients in the office on a nonstop assembly line. Increasing numbers of them want a nine-to-five job and more free time on nights and weekends. At the same time, they hope for patient compliance and loyalty while acknowledging diminished expectations of their own roles as professional caretakers.

The field of primary care now proposes a solution like the "medical home" concept to provide higher reimbursements and prestige for the field. This approach involves emphasizing the patient perspective more in delivering care.

Yet, the medical home approach does not acknowledge what many medical students and residents increasingly believe about primary care, whether it is indeed true or not, that in any form the work involved is more chaotic and less intellectually stimulating than almost any other specialty, and can never match the better salaries and lifestyles afforded by specialties such as dermatology, radiology, or ophthalmology. And even when the work is perceived as interesting by would-be physicians, many of them flinch at the breadth of knowledge needed to become a competent primary care doctor, opting instead to become masters of narrow specialty areas.

It was not always this way. Up until the 1970s, generalist medicine, the forerunner of today's primary care, was held in high esteem by physicians, medical students, insurers, and the general public. Whereas contemporary television shows such as *ER*, *House*, and *Grey's Anatomy* shape our perception of the "best" and "coolest" doctors as superspecialists interacting with one another within hospital settings that are fast-paced, exciting, and attractively quirky, and where many diagnoses are made magically through the sheer brilliance and eccentricities of the physicians involved, it was an older, compassionate family physician named Marcus Welby who glorified the generalist physician's role in the 1970s.

Welby was a veteran practitioner devoted less to magic bullets and more to exploring in-depth his patients' many problems, from the physical to psychological. An admired detective in his job, mentoring younger doctors, Welby used his general medicine skills, years of experience, and ability to relate to his patients to solve a full range of clinical mysteries each and every week. The tools in his arsenal were not technology or superspecialist knowledge but commonsense approaches that involved listening to patients, taking histories, and gaining understanding of how the aspects of a patient's life fit together to drive his or her symptoms. Welby sought to know and have relationships with his patients, understand the psychosocial backdrops for their illnesses, and through this connection he had the key to successful diagnosis and treatment.

Most doctors these days are not Marcus Welby, most medical students do not wish to become Marcus Welby, and insurance companies do not pay for the qualities typified by Welby's approach to care. No longer does the wise, all-knowing primary care physician grab the attention of television viewers. Outpatient care, with its low-tech but effective tools, does not attract viewers or medical students the same way as in-your-face life and death struggles. In the early twenty-first century, taking a good family history or preventing a disease ten years before it would hit a patient does not sell to a viewing audience like an organ transplant or car wreck.

Ironically, many patients increasingly need the Welby-type practitioner and the medicine practiced by that practitioner, given their own unhealthiness and a health care system with little patience for prevention or promoting healthier lives. The primary care setting is where the vast majority of those who suffer from chronic diseases like diabetes and hypertension get their care. It is where most of us go first when something is wrong with us, or when we simply want to learn how to get healthier. Primary care doctors are the doctors we trust because we see and share with them the most.

In theory, primary care is about treating the patient as a whole person—a living, breathing organism with a specific lifestyle, work and home environment, and biological risk profile. PCPs are the doctors trained to see us in this holistic way. While they provide a lot of low-level health care, their importance in making us feel better cannot be underestimated. They get us to accept that nothing serious is wrong when we feel ill. They are the ones who first care for our children, treat our run-of-the-mill infections, prevent future illness, help correct our lives to lessen the effects of chronic disease, and often first diagnose serious conditions. Though not trained or paid formally to do it, they are usually the first professionals who identify depression, stress, and sadness in many of our lives. In these ways, PCPs are the foot soldiers of medicine. They are the low-paid grunts defending the front lines of the health care delivery system from hordes of sicker people. They are often the last line of defense against unnecessary, expensive care and a system that divides patients into discrete parts attended to in an impersonal manner.

The Need for a Strong Primary Care System

Current, unarguable realities support the conclusion that we need a stronger primary care system staffed by doctors who are generalists, listeners, confidantes, and care coordinators. These realities include rising rates of chronic diseases such as obesity, diabetes, and heart disease; longer life spans; the greater attention now given to prevention to stabilize health care costs, deal with chronic diseases effectively, and increase the quality of life for all citizens; and a renewed focus in the United States on health care reform, in particular providing more citizens with health insurance and access to basic primary care through a medical home.

Estimates show that up to 50 percent of the U.S. population has a chronic medical condition. Fifty percent of this group has multiple chronic conditions. Two-thirds of these individuals are over the age of sixty-five. Two-thirds of all adult Americans are either overweight or obese. The prevalence of obesity over the past three decades has more than doubled among adults age twenty to seventy-four, from 15 to 33 percent.[1] Nineteen percent of children (age six to eleven) and 17 percent of adolescents (age twelve to nineteen) were overweight in 2003, and we can project a significant number of potentially obese adults in the near future.[2]

These statistics call for a strong primary care workforce. Obesity leads to greater prevalence of chronic diseases like hypertension and diabetes. It is a condition that cannot be cured with a single prescription, doctor's visit, or procedure. It requires extended consultation, monitoring, and significant adjustments in lifestyle. It requires doctors who know the patients and appreciate what is possible with respect to lifestyle, nutritional, and attitudinal adjustments. It demands proactive prevention strategies that involve physical activity, diet modifications, and in some instances, extended pharmacological or psychological interventions. More overweight and obese individuals in American society mean increased numbers of visits to primary care offices, a greater need for prevention and counseling by PCPs, and a less healthy general population that suffers from a range of illnesses simultaneously. Millions of overweight and obese children place a greater strain on the primary care pediatric system.

One third of all Americans suffer from cardiovascular disease.[3] The more common forms of this disease are hypertension and coronary artery disease, conditions not immediately life threatening but requiring constant monitoring and prevention-related activities. Most nonsurgical services for hypertension and heart disease are provided by primary care, which is a cost-efficient level of care. Over seventy million outpatient visits to doctors' offices in 2004 were for patients with a primary diagnosis of cardiovascular disease.[4] Avoiding emergent situations like stroke or heart attack, respiratory distress, and high blood pressure involves extensive involvement by a patient's PCP in medication monitoring, diet and exercise counseling, and regular testing. And heart disease does not affect only the very old. Over 60 percent of those with the disease are younger than sixty-five.[5] This means that many people will be living with heart disease for years to come, and making visits to the primary care office.

Diabetes is the third player in the twenty-first century chronic disease troika that demands more services from the field of primary care. Ten percent of people over the age of twenty in the United States have diabetes, or close to 20 million individuals.[6] In 2005, there were one and a half million new cases, the majority of which occurred in the relatively young forty to fifty-nine age group. Diabetes is more prevalent among individuals sixty years and older, meaning that more new cases will occur as people live longer.[7] Over $100 billion dollars annually gets spent on diabetes care.[8] Diabetes is a manageable disease that with the right treatment and attention does not have to significantly lessen quality of life. Yet death rates are rising, especially for younger citizens.[9]

This grim statistic is despite the fact that we go to the doctor's office 27 million times a year for diabetes care alone. All those visits—and over 70,000 individuals still die from this chronic disease annually.[10] PCPs are needed to help prevent diabetic complications through active preventive strategies involving nutrition and exercise, as well as monitoring of blood pressure, renal function, blood glucose, blood lipids, and eyesight. More overweight and obese children at present will cause a significant increase in the prevalence of Type II diabetes over the next twenty years in the young adult population. The fact remains: primary care is the first line of defense in managing diabetes. It is also the first line of defense in preventing diabetes in patients who have what is called impaired fasting glucose or impaired glucose tolerance, precursors to the disease and present in anywhere from 40 to 55 million Americans.[11]

The declining health of many Americans, including those in the more affluent middle class, is not limited to conditions such as cardiovascular disease and diabetes. PCPs diagnose and treat other major diseases in large numbers as well. For example, over a quarter of adult Americans suffer from a diagnosable mental disorder in any given year.[12] Nearly half of this group will have two or more mental-health diagnoses with which to contend at a given time.[13] Depression is the leading cause of illness in the United States for individuals age fifteen to forty-four, and affects almost 7 percent of the general population.[14] It is the primary care system that often acts as the initial intake and care point for patients with mental health disorders. For some, the primary care system acts as the only point of care for treating their behavioral health problems.

Older Patients, Prevention, and Health Care Reform

Our average life expectancy is now almost seventy-eight years, a record level, ten years higher than in 1970, and as high as most other countries in the world.[15] In addition, the first wave of 80 million baby boomers is reaching retirement age. Living longer produces an increased demand for all health care services, but particularly for primary care. Individuals sixty-five years of age and older tend to see their doctors two to three times more often than younger individuals.[16] This group is more likely to suffer age-related chronic diseases like arthritis, and have minor complaints that involve the heart, mobility, and respiratory and digestive systems. They are more likely to need medication regimens checked regularly, as well as common clinical indicators like blood pressure and cholesterol. They also need immunizations, mammograms, prostate exams, endoscopies, and colonoscopies at higher rates than the general population.[17] All of these procedures are done either directly or, as is the case now, coordinated by the primary care physician.

There is a growing emphasis on prevention in the United States. But to do prevention right requires that PCPs spend a lot of time with individual patients in their exam rooms. PCPs provide over 85 percent of all the preventive care visits in the United States.[18] One recent study estimated that simply to comply with existing national prevention guidelines for adults and children would require seven hours out of each PCP's day.[19] Seven hours for prevention alone. No PCP has seven hours available daily for preventive care. Still, this soft mandate for preventive medicine emphasizes how much PCPs are needed if our country is to lower health care costs by avoiding more acute diseases, producing healthier citizens, and increasing the quality of care in the system. There are no shortcuts when it comes to prevention.

Finally, there is health care reform. The focus currently is on providing all citizens with some form or basic health insurance, developing a stronger primary care system in the United States, and emphasizing preventive care and chronic disease management in order to limit costs and improve the quality of life for all citizens. Within this debate, the concept of the medical home has been put forth as a means by which to center the basic elements of preventive care and care coordination within the purview of the primary care physician's office.[20] The medical home concept has found traction within the primary care physician community and by employers interested in reducing their health care costs while still improving quality of care for their employees.

The tenets of a medical home involve not-so-new ideas related to care management, adopting a "whole person" orientation to care, convenient access to primary care doctors for patients, the use of evidence-based practices for prevention and chronic disease management, and one-to-one physician-patient relationships. There is growing recognition that only a strong primary care system will allow for proper implementation of the medical home concept. There is also acknowledgment that if more people have health insurance, the existing primary care system will not be able to handle the increased demand. Health reform makes maintaining a strong primary care system a critical policy issue. To provide people with insurance coverage and then no accessible system of basic, primary care undermines the country's effort to make people healthier.

The Decline of Generalist Medicine in the United States

Until the 1980s, few people understood the term "primary care." Proposed in the 1960s, it sought to clarify the importance and role of generalist medicine in an advancing era of technologically driven, specialty care.[21] In its 1996 report entitled "Primary Care: America's Health in a New Era," the Institute of Medicine (IOM), the nation's premier health advisory body, defined primary care as "the provision of integrated, accessible, health care services by clinicians who are accountable for addressing a large majority of personal health care needs, developing a sustained partnership with patients, and practicing in the context of the family and the community."[22]

The IOM emphasized the diversity and breadth inherent in the definition of this term, stressing that primary care included "the care provided by certain clinicians," "a set of activities," "a level of care or setting," "a set of attributes" for care, and "a strategy for organizing the health care system."[23] In using this expansive definition, the field of primary care now attempts to compete alongside specialty medicine. But the overt marketing of generalist care through national definitions was not needed three decades ago.

Until the 1980s, defining what primary care consisted of was irrelevant. People receiving health care in the United States knew only one type of physician well, and that was their generalist doctor, the forerunner of today's primary care doctor. At the time, advances in fields such as surgery, cardiology, orthopedics, and radiology had begun to spur a revolution in medical care practice that would reshape payment systems, patient expectations, the physician and larger healthcare workforce, and care delivery. But before that, individuals and their families went to their neighborhood primary care doctor exclusively when they felt a doctor's visit was necessary. This physician was not someone trained in one specific medical field whose job involved singular treatment of a specific patient problem. Instead, it was someone whose everyday work involved practicing across many different clinical areas of expertise and attending to a full range of patient complaints and conditions.

The generalist physician of the past knew patients over long stretches of time, held their trust to make health care decisions for them, and handled a large, diverse scope of work. In a time before urgent care centers, retail medical clinics, and direct patient contact with specialists like orthopedists, the generalist practice was one-stop shopping for individuals and their illnesses. These doctors often worked alone or in very small groups, owned their practices, were well known in the local community, and served as the central hub for connecting select patients with different specialists on the rarer occasions when clinical cases grew too complex.

A typical generalist practice in the 1960s or 1970s was located in a neighborhood house or apartment suite, perhaps in a small office building, and staffed with a physician or two, a supporting nurse, and perhaps one or two clerical staff. Records, notes, and billing were all done by paper; there were few

outside demands for data on how doctors did their work; and all patient information remained within the confines of the practice, under the direct control of
the physician. It was paternalistic in both the best and worst ways, with the
generalist physician telling the patient what to do, and expecting complete
compliance with his orders.

The scope of work for generalist doctors during this time was full and
varied. Generalists oversaw the care of their patients in the hospital from
admission to discharge, performed after-hours call duties to address patient
emergencies that required several or more nights per week of interruptions and
decreased sleep, visited patients when they went to hospital emergency rooms,
and performed different procedures on patients in their offices. In every sense,
patients were the clinical property of the generalist, loaned out to other specialists in the hospital when that generalist felt additional episodic care was
needed, but returned to the generalist once that care was over. Specialists knew
this, and relied on the generalist to refer patients to them. This relationship
gave the generalist power and encouraged specialists to interact and get to
know the generalists in their community. Patients could see one physician and
feel like that physician knew their full range of medical needs.

Like all medical specialties of that era, generalist medicine was dominated
by middle- and upper-middle-class white men who worked long hours and on
weekends, cared about being successful businessmen as well as physicians,
and saw their families less as a result. In return for this commitment to building a profitable business and meeting patient demand, generalist doctors got
paid in accordance with what their usual and customary rates were for the time
and services they and their local primary care colleagues provided. There were
only one or two insurance companies with whom to deal, and these companies
rarely questioned physician decisions. A forty-five-minute patient visit could
be billed and reimbursed in ways decided by the generalist, and payment
moved in tandem with the idiosyncratic practice patterns of the local generalist community.

Office visits between doctor and patient lasted as long as the doctor preferred. There was no time limit for a patient visit. Doctors were reimbursed for
longer time spent with the patient, regardless of the diagnosis or services rendered, as long as other physicians in the community billed similarly. There was
no set number of patients to see in a given day to generate adequate practice
reimbursement, because the volume of individual visits was not the deciding
factor in how much PCPs could get compensated.

Adequate reimbursement came from whatever the physician felt was billable that day to meet his own definition of quality care and make ends meet. If

ten forty-five-minute visits did the trick, then there was nothing wrong with conducting longer visits where time was spent talking with the patient and the social interaction was extensive. Waiting rooms were rarely filled, the physician often ducked out during the day to go to the hospital or an outside meeting, and the typical practice functioned in a more leisurely manner. The workday sped up or slowed down at the sole discretion of generalist doctors: what they felt like doing, the types of patients with whom they wanted to spend more time, and how much money they wanted to make.

To assure adequate work variety, generalist physicians moved around during their workday, going to the hospital each morning and evening to see patients, participating on hospital committees, interacting with specialists in the community at hospital events and medical association meetings, and making emergency house calls. This work supplemented an office-based schedule that involved performing procedures such as splinting, casting, and stitching, basic acute care, and some chronic disease care.

Generalist doctors could engage in this wide array of duties because payers and patients alike assumed that they were trained and experienced enough to handle many clinical situations. A quality movement and technological revolution that would justify having specialized doctors assume direct care over parts of their work had not yet begun. No one looked over the doctor's shoulder. Patients went to generalists for everything, were managed by generalists through their serious illnesses, and insurers paid generalists adequately for attending to whatever patient needs the doctors deemed reasonable. This did not mean patients received the highest-quality, most cost-effective care from the generalist. It meant only that generalists were perceived as the appropriate caregivers for a wide scope of clinical problems.

Of course, care for all conditions was simpler back then. For example, diabetic care consisted not of the tens of pages of care guidelines now followed but of three basic procedures: regular blood glucose checks, proper management of insulin therapy, and patient physical exams. The contributing roles of patient education and self-management, proper diet, physical activity, as well as proper physician management of other conditions such as heart disease and high blood pressure were not yet well understood and not part of the generalist's approach to managing diabetes. Usually less than a handful of available drug options were available for every clinical situation, ranging from respiratory and sinus infections to controlling lipids and cholesterol, thus making the choices of what to prescribe easier. Fewer patients had multiple chronic diseases that interacted with one another to create highly complex care situations. If a generalist faced an uncertain diagnosis in a patient, he or she could admit that patient to the local hospital without questioning from insurance companies. Specialists would help identify the problem, treat it if necessary, and then return that patient to the management of the generalist.

The more glamorous current-day physician view reflected on television provides no room for the typical office-based primary care physician of today, yet it is shows such as *ER* and *Grey's Anatomy* that medical students watch religiously to learn about the work of their profession.[24] The PCP is no longer perceived as the "all knowing" physician within medicine, no longer sees patients in the hospital or does procedures, performs less and less complex acute care, deals with sicker, less compliant patients, faces packed waiting rooms, and remains in the office the entire work day, socially isolated from hospital and specialist colleagues, in order to bill enough visits for adequate pay.

We now perceive that the best and brightest physicians are found in the hospital, moving around effortlessly and engaging in a never-ending routine of intellectual foreplay while doing narrowly defined clinical work rather than expansive primary care. It is in the television-constructed hospital where complex life-and-death decisions are made matter-of-factly, where diseases meet their match through the application of other-worldly intelligence and cutting-edge technology, and where patients are not so much human beings as containment vessels for interesting and hard-to-identify pathologies.

While selling the hospital setting and specialists as the appropriate purveyors of "real" medicine is the core message of these popular shows, they more simply reflect a larger reality that has played out in the U.S. health care system over the past few decades. That reality is the rendering of generalist medicine to secondary status among insurers, medical specialties, medical students, and patients. Society has shunned primary care and primary care physicians. The result has been a shrinking primary care workforce, the transfer of traditional primary care work from generalists to specialists, the rise of alternative forms of primary care, and a new business model of primary care delivery that deemphasizes both the spirit and substance of the definition of primary care suggested by the Institute of Medicine. Ironically, these changes have occurred while the country's demand for generalist medicine and the Welby-type doctor grows, creating a perfect storm for crisis in our health care system.

The Supply–Demand Tensions in Primary Care

Today's PCPs are grouped into three categories: general internists, family physicians, and general pediatricians. Some also categorize geriatricians and obstetrician-gynecologists (OB/GYNs) as primary care physicians, but there are few geriatricians around these days, and OB/GYNs are surgeons and reproductive specialists first and foremost. At the turn of the twentieth century, 85 percent of all doctors were considered "primary" or "general" care. In the early 1960s, this figure was down to half of all doctors in the United States. Now, in the early twenty-first century, PCPs represent a third of the physician workforce.[25]

This shrinking proportion of PCPs in the total medical workforce is likely to get worse. For example, between 1996 and 2007, U.S. medical school graduates choosing family medicine decreased by more than 50 percent, to 8 percent of all U.S. medical school graduates.[26] It is estimated that less than 20 percent of all physicians who began residency in 2005 will practice as generalists. A recent survey of medical students going into internal medicine residencies identified less than 2 percent who said they would go into primary care.[27] Instead, increasing numbers of internal medicine and pediatric residents are choosing to subspecialize in a narrow field rather than practice generalist medicine. Fewer general primary care residency positions are being made available, and fewer still are being filled with graduates from U.S. medical schools.[28] For example, less than half of recent residents entering family medicine graduated from U.S. medical schools.[29]

Many areas of the United States now suffer from a lack of availability of primary care physicians. Rural areas, inner cities, and even middle-class suburbs increasingly do not seem to have enough of these practitioners. More than 20 million Americans live in nonmetropolitan areas with a shortage of PCPs.[30] The increased demand for primary care services expected to occur because of an aging population, population growth, heightened focus on prevention, and the increased incidence of chronic disease in the general population may require between 20 to 30 percent more primary care physicians by the year 2020.[31]

Overall, U.S. statistics show that the number of ambulatory care office visits went up by 31 percent, to over one billion total visits, between 1994 and 2004, due to increases in population and in health service utilization per person.[32] Primary care office visits made up almost half of that one billion visit total.[33] Successful health care reform, both at the state and federal levels, could add to the problem by increasing demand for primary care. For example, after implementing its universal health insurance mandate, the state of Massachusetts found that the primary care physician infrastructure was insufficient to handle the expected added services for individuals who now had insurance.[34] At the same time as demand is growing for primary care, the percentage of U.S. medical school graduates choosing a primary care specialty is decreasing, and an increasing percentage of physicians nationally are moving toward retirement age.[35]

This tension between primary care supply and demand has not materialized overnight. The topic has been overanalyzed statistically by professional associations, politicians, health advocates, and academics. There is little doubt that the specialization movement in medicine generally, and in primary care particularly, has greatly undermined the appeal of generalist primary care careers. The preference of many medical students to pursue a nonprimary care specialty like orthopedics or radiology instead of primary care has existed for some time. These specialties always pay more, often a lot more, and are perceived as more prestigious and intellectually challenging. But conventional wisdom says that money is the big lure. For example, the average orthopedic surgeon makes over $400,000 annually and the average radiologist does similarly well.[36]

While these specialties draw mostly from medical students who are not interested in primary care, the trend toward primary care subspecialization is newer and more alarming. It diverts many students who are also interested in generalist primary care. Primary care subspecialization is different from a generalist primary care field in the lower intensity of the "first contact, longitudinality, coordination, and comprehensiveness" of the patient care provided.[37] It focuses on specific conditions or disease states rather than the entire patient or his or her general condition over time. It does not concern itself as much with prevention or continuity of care as with curing acute problems episodically already affecting the patient. Examples of primary care subspecializations include cardiology (heart), nephrology (kidneys), and gastroenterology (digestive system), and these may be either child or adult focused.

The primary care subspecialization trend is highlighted in a published study from 2005. This study included almost all of the third-year internal medicine residents in the United States, surveyed annually from 1998 to 2003.[38] The percentage of residents stating that they intended to pursue a general internal medicine career shrunk from 54 to 27 percent from the 1998 to the 2003 third-year class. On the other hand, the percentage intending to go into an internal medicine subspecialty increased over the same time period from 42 to 57 percent. In addition, in this same study only 19 percent of internal medicine residents just beginning their residencies in 2003 intended to pursue a work career in general internal medicine, compared to 46 percent of first-year residents in 1998.[39]

A second study also published in 2005 showed the continued desire of medical students to go into specialty care. It included 97 percent of all active residents in the United States, and found that the percentage of total family medicine residency program slots (a generalist PCP field) occupied by U.S.

medical school graduates dropped from 78 to 51 percent between 1995 and 2005.[40] This trend continued into 2007, with only about 42 percent of the available family medicine positions filled by U.S. medical graduates.[41] Since 1997, the number of medical students choosing family medicine has declined over 50 percent.[42] This growing lack of demand has contributed to a shrinking in the number of available residency positions in family medicine, from 2,941 in 1995 to 2,621 in 2007.[43]

The "match rates" for internal medicine and pediatrics, along with family medicine, are substantially lower than for other medical specialties where U.S. medical graduates are concerned.[44] For example, in 2007 internal medicine residency positions were filled by U.S. graduates only 57 percent of the time, and for pediatrics 73 percent. Compared to orthopedic surgery (94 percent), radiology (89 percent), otolaryngology (93 percent), anesthesiology (78 percent), and emergency medicine (80 percent), it is clear that generalist primary care looks less and less appealing to the U.S. graduate.[45]

The acceptance of primary care subspecialization within the medical profession is witnessed in the fact that subspecialty residency programs are growing nationally, while generalist primary care residency programs shrink.[46] This is a disturbing trend, and implies that the medical profession contributes to the problem by creating more of these niche residency programs to meet demand, rather than trying to restrict supply. As a result, a troubling chicken-and-egg dynamic plays out: fewer students choose primary care residencies, so fewer primary care residency positions are made available. As these positions shrink, medical students perceive primary care at best as a struggling, downsizing area of medicine, and at worst a dead-end career more appropriate as the consolation prize when attempts to get into higher-prestige specialty residencies fail.

The Rise of Primary Care Alternatives

Physician assistants (PAs) and nurse practitioners (NPs) are filling the void resulting from current supply-demand tensions in primary care. Ironically, both groups were formed in the 1960s to address primary care physician shortages in underserved areas and because of new public insurance programs such as Medicare and Medicaid. Both of these groups are expanding to meet the demand for delivering primary care services within a business model driven by the need for face-to-face patient visits in order to get paid. With the declining attractiveness of primary care careers for aspiring physicians, both PAs and NPs represent viable competition for sizable portions of lower-complexity primary care services. For example, they have been shown to provide similar care across a wide array of conditions to PCPs in terms of both costs and quality.[47] They also receive high marks for patient satisfaction when providing primary care, in some cases higher than their physician counterparts.[48]

PAs and NPs have evolved under the support and supervision of the primary care physician community. This has meant formal PCP oversight of their work, limitations on their scope of practice, and annual salaries that are approximately half on average compared to primary care specialties like general internal medicine and family medicine. The typical full-time NP and PA earns approximately $75,000 annually. As human capital that may substitute for PCPs in a variety of care circumstances, both groups increase the profitability of a typical primary care practice. For example, each patient visit that an NP or PA conducts in place of a PCP can provide increased net revenue because of the smaller provider salaries involved in the visit itself, since insurance reimbursements for NP and PA visits in many situations are only slightly less than for PCP visits. This relative cost advantage is a primary reason for the continuing growth of these two occupations. There are over 200,000 NPs and PAs in total in the United States, and both groups have grown or are expected to grow 20 percent or more in the early part of this century.

PCPs are complicit in the promotion of NPs and PAs as viable alternatives to much of the basic primary care they now provide, the bulk of which includes common acute illnesses and less complex chronic disease management. Faced with decreasing profit margins in their practices, PCPs employ NPs and PAs as a strategic response to remaining financially viable in the marketplace. As a business decision, it makes sense. However, the longer-term effect on primary care physicians as an occupational group is more complex to assess. For instance, if NPs and PAs provide equivalent care in some instances, is this justification enough to allow them to practice primary care completely independently from PCPs, perhaps through businesses they own and control?

One point of view is that the longer such providers practice without discernable differences compared to PCPs, the stronger the case made for their ability to assume equal control over a meaningful portion of primary care work. A contrasting perspective says that PCPs have more training and experience than these other providers, and while the latter are appropriate for lower-level primary care situations, the former are necessary for the delivery of complex primary care. Regardless, through their heavy involvement at present in delivering basic acute care and chronic disease management, NPs and PAs grow increasingly familiar to patients as competent occupational groups that can get the job done.

Besides the occupational groups who are assuming prominence in the transformation of primary care delivery, the traditional primary care practice faces future competition from alternative delivery sites such as urgent care centers and retail clinics. These settings are a direct threat to the traditional primary care practice for specific types of primary care services. These settings also rely upon nonphysician providers such as NPs and PAs rather than PCPs to deliver significant portions of the care. Urgent care centers have been around for several decades, and approximately eight thousand of them exist in the United States. These are settings in which much of the clinical work consists of common acute care illness and easy-to-treat emergency conditions. Urgent care centers are popular because patients may be unable to get timely appointments for these types of emergency conditions in the traditional primary care practice they use. For patients without a regular PCP, which these days are many, urgent care centers offer a trusted, stable source of care with low barriers to entry.

Convenience, speed, and price are the main reasons why retail clinics have gained popularity over the past few years. As a newer phenomenon in primary care, they seek to carve out a market niche in providing patients with a limited array of cheaper health care services that include treatment for common acute illnesses, health promotion activities such as physicals and screenings, basic laboratory testing, and immunizations.[49] Retail clinics are walk-in clinical delivery sites embedded within larger retail stores such as Wal-Mart and CVS. There are now almost one thousand of them in the United States, and it is anticipated that their numbers may grow to over five thousand over the next several years.[50] Similar to urgent care centers, they provide flexible hours of operation, including evenings and weekends, do not require appointments, and are intended to move the patient through the visit in a brief time period.

Almost half of consumers in a recent survey said they would have little issue with receiving care at a retail clinic staffed by NPs and not PCPs.[51] While the clinical services offered in such settings are narrowly defined, they appear to meet a need for young adult patients, patients without regular sources of primary care, and patients who do not have insurance. A recent study found that retail clinics served a higher than average percentage of patients falling into these three categories.[52] In addition, patients appear satisfied with the care they receive in these settings, the settings have high visibility in the community, and they provide a level of convenience and speed that meets expectations and rivals or exceeds that which traditional primary care offices can provide.[53]

Basic, low-complexity primary care services are the bailiwick of these new delivery structures. This same study found that ten clinical problems falling into the categories described above accounted for almost all of the services provided in over one million retail clinic visit instances, compared to less than 15 percent of adult PCP and 30 percent of pediatric PCP visits.[54] This means that PCPs working in traditional primary care offices deal with clinical problems on a vastly broader, diverse scale than do retail clinics. Primary care offices, despite the growth of retail clinics, remain the most sophisticated, complete sources of care for patients, especially in the areas of chronic disease management and behavioral health care—two areas where rising demand is seen nationally. They also are the only viable primary care settings that can provide continuous care for patients with chronic conditions.

But what cannot be understated is that retail clinics provide basic, affordable primary care service delivery that is easily accessed and quickly performed. They serve a primary clientele that does not have allegiance to a particular PCP or primary care office, and one that might otherwise not pursue care without the clinic's presence. As a result, retail clinics will continue to fill service gaps that traditional primary care offices and PCPs have an increasingly difficult time filling, given large numbers of existing patients who clog the daily schedules, and the need to generate larger reimbursements from individual patient visits to cover the higher costs of physician-based care. They may also contribute to the shifting perception of generalist medicine within our society from a relationship-oriented brand of total care to a transaction-oriented series of compartmentalized visits that involve routine care. Ironically, it is the manner in which PCPs now work within their traditional office settings more than anything else that furthers this perceptual shift.

The Dysfunctional Primary Care Business Model

The halcyon days of generalist care, where PCPs alone determined the scope, substance, and economic value of all primary work has been replaced by an environment in which PCPs must make serious choices about which work to keep, which to jettison, and how to maintain job and patient satisfaction within a rigidly imposed reimbursement model that favors quick episodic care. The twenty-first-century U.S. health care system now pays PCPs less for the same type of care, ignores the practice of cognitive medicine that involves skills such as history taking and counseling, demands that PCPs see lots of patients in a given day to breakeven, motivates PCPs to give up low-margin parts of their business regardless of the personal or patient-related benefits derived from having PCPs engaged in that business, and increasingly buys the notion that other medical specialists are better suited to perform the more complex aspects of traditional generalist work such as different types of procedures and hospital medicine.

For most types of primary care, the fifteen-minute visit is now the normative standard. In the early twenty-first century, PCPs are professional piece-rate workers in the sense that they are paid on the basis that a face-to-face patient visit actually occurs, and less on what actually happens during that visit (that is, the actual diagnosis treated or addressed). Where the generalist of 1970 could spend forty-five minutes talking with a patient and be paid for that time, now insurers affix precise dollar amounts and time limits to different clinical diagnoses. This leaves PCPs little discretion to make their own judgments about whether or not more time is needed with a particular patient. But it also does not mean that the generalist's judgment about how much time to spend with patients in 1970 was good medicine. A forty-five-minute visit might have been unnecessary for treating the patient appropriately and may simply have been a way to generate adequate income without having to see too many patients in a given day.

PCPs spend the majority of their day in direct patient care. One recent survey found that the mean number of daily patients seen by a PCP was twenty-nine.[55] Almost all of them now spend a full day in the office setting, no longer doing work in the hospital, making house calls, or performing nonrevenue-generating activities such as committee work, at least during normal work hours. They cannot take time to do these other things. The typical workday of a primary care physician in the early twenty-first century is built on seeing as many patients as possible in the office in a given day.

Since fewer and fewer PCPs do procedures such as injections, biopsies, and cardiac stress tests in their offices, almost all of the primary care revenue within a practice now comes from reimbursement provided by the patient visit. Insurers financially motivate PCPs to keep patient visits brief. For example, a PCP may bill for visits that involve varying levels of complexity or length, but the relative additional dollars associated with complex or longer visits often does not justify the extra time and expertise needed relative to the simpler visit. In other words, it can be more profitable for a PCP to see four established, generally healthy patients who have basic acute problems in the course of an hour than seeing two established, sicker patients who require extended visits for services related to managing their chronic diseases. If patients have multiple issues, which many do, often the PCP cannot bill for treating both diagnoses in the same encounter but instead must bring the patient back for separate visits to address each of the issues in a way that provides adequate reimbursement.

This emphasis on both speed and numbers raises tensions in the practice of today's primary care medicine; tensions that never existed for the generalist of 1970. For example, as greater numbers of patients with behavioral health issues present in the PCP's office, and the PCP's reimbursement system is not set up to pay them adequately for this type of care, PCPs have four suboptimal choices before them: either attempt to provide appropriate care by spending time with the patient, thereby sacrificing other office visits and earning less money for the practice; attempt to provide more complex behavioral medicine within the confines of fifteen- or twenty-minute visits that may produce low-quality care; offer "quick-and-dirty" prescription therapies to patients; or refer patients to behavioral health specialists who are in short supply causing delays of weeks or months before they are seen. It is often left up to individual PCPs to resolve this tension, and as a result the choice itself, made many times for patients over the course of a work week, can undermine the physician's job satisfaction.

It is now also more accepted from a quality-of-care perspective that PCPs are not as appropriate for doing complex office procedures like colonoscopies and stress tests as gastroenterologists and cardiologists, for example. Instead, the argument goes, this type of work should be left to these specialists who do high numbers of procedures on a regular basis. Low-level procedures such as splinting sprained limbs or joints, or wound debridement and stitching, also now succumb to the whims of patients who may believe going to an urgent care center, emergency room, or specialist is faster and higher quality. And specialists desire to do as many of these simpler procedures as possible, since they pay well compared to the basic office visits in which they might engage with patients.

Most primary care practices now entrust care of their hospitalized patients to a new group of physicians called "hospitalists." The growth of hospital medicine as a separate specialty has accelerated over the past ten years. Since 1994, over 12,000 physicians nationally have taken up hospital medicine as a career field. It is the fastest-growing specialty in medicine, with the potential for over double the current number by 2010. Ironically, many of the doctors making hospital medicine a flourishing field would likely have been office based PCPs if the choice to become hospitalists had not been there. Three-quarters of hospitalists are trained in general internal medicine, and approximately another 15 percent in family practice or general pediatrics.

The need for hospitalists derives from the increased complexity of hospital medicine, combined with the economic realities of both hospital medicine and primary care today. Hospital reimbursement for primary care physicians is low. In addition, overall inpatient volume for the typical PCP at any given time is much less than in 1970 because of the health care system's enhanced ability to care for patients outside of the hospital and reimbursement incentives that encourage keeping patients in the ambulatory setting. As a result, PCPs earn greater reimbursement seeing patients in the outpatient setting during the same couple hours it might take to visit one or a few patients in the hospital. As PCPs do less and less hospital medicine, the appropriate standard of care from a quality point of view is that they do not perform this type of work but instead hand it over to the hospitalists who spend all day, every day doing nothing but caring for hospitalized patients.

These shifts in the work PCPs now perform, how they adapt to their work and get it done, and what it means for the workers and primary care are key foci in this book. For example, as PCPs have accommodated a reimbursement model that rewards speed over substance, how do they manage the demands imposed by sicker patients coming into their offices for care? For the multitude of patients with chronic diseases or behavioral health issues, are PCPs able to employ the necessary communication, listening, and history-taking skills in large enough quantities to produce high-quality care? Do PCPs enjoy practicing in daily environments where the work variety is lessened? What type of primary care field are patients left with after years of a business model where key services get financially undervalued, and the key knowledge workers providing these services adapt in ways that allow them to excel at completing customer transactions rather than building patient relationships?

Knowing More about the Everyday Experience of Primary Care Physicians

Anecdotes abound about the increasingly hectic, unsatisfying nature of primary care workdays across all types of settings, and about the dissatisfaction of primary care physicians. But to understand the current transformation of this field better, and how PCPs think and act within the transformation to shape primary care's future, we should know more about the everyday experience of being a primary care physician.

All workers make choices in adapting to developments thrust upon them. Work is restructured, sacrificed, and its pace modified by the individuals engaged in it. This is done to preserve control, income, prestige, and job satisfaction. But trade-offs are made by the workers themselves. For example, certain forms of autonomy get prioritized at the expense of lesser "luxuries" such as job variety and intellectual stimulation. In a primary care system where patient demand rises, and the business model rewards volume, PCPs engage work in a more transactional manner.

Pressures to meet production targets, in the form of patients walking through the door each day, require PCPs increasingly to emphasize the economic rather than social aspects of the customer encounter. Patients become "consumers" or "customers" and the interactions with doctors grow ever more businesslike, streamlined, and impersonal. The drive to standardize, divide up labor, make work simpler, and pursue economies of scale in how things are done becomes a rational, expected motivator of behavior in a transactional system, which in turn shifts the expectations and values PCPs bring to their jobs.

This study fills an important gap by exploring, from the perspectives of a variety of primary care physicians, the ways in which the field of primary care is adapting to developments affecting it. Extant literature has focused sharply on the developments themselves, and on external market responses such as the development of new occupational groups and primary care delivery structures. But much less attention has been paid to how individual doctors "in the trenches" are now coping with the everyday world around them. This sociological exploration can inform larger policy questions that relate to issues such as how to promote primary care to future generations of medical students, how best to intervene now in enhancing the experiences of existing PCPs and their patients, and what type of work and decision making should be advocated as purviews of primary care doctors and their traditional practice settings.

For example, most of the present discussion about the appropriate core of future primary care work and identity centers on the medical home concept, a concept envisioned by primary care professional associations as the means by which to reassert the primary care physician's importance and leadership role in the medical hierarchy. Through implementation of the medical home, PCPs would gain back formal recognition, through added payment, as care coordinators, overseers of health promotion and disease prevention in the clinical setting, and first-contact professionals that patients access first for care. NPs and PAs would be part of the "physician-led" team, but PCPs would retain the mantle of leadership in primary care settings. The traditional primary care office would be the legitimate focus for a patient's medical home, with emerging structures such as retail clinics providing supplemental basic care subservient to the care provided in the traditional PCP office.

The technical, idealistic vision of the medical home as a savior for primary care cannot be fulfilled if PCPs find themselves in an everyday work setting where patient demand is still not easily controlled or predicted, where they are still forced to refer patients out quicker to specialists because of time or reimbursement constraints, where they are not adequately prepared for certain types of care, or in which their own scope of work still narrows toward an emphasis on highly routine, less complex care. These realities have already modified the way in which many PCPs think about their careers, clinical skills, and patients. And such modifications may not easily conform to what will be asked of them and their work in a medical-home role.

As a result, additional changes are needed beyond the much talked about reimbursement increases for PCPs or technological enhancements to make the medical-home model work. These additional changes once again involve transforming the social and psychological dynamics associated with physician-patient interactions in primary care. PCPs will have to readapt in thought and action to a workplace built not only on high-volume medicine but now also on care management and coordination. They will have to embrace new work and work roles, and think of other staff and patients in different ways. Yet having moved through one major form of adaptation over the past twenty years, in negotiating and making the best of a transactional business model in which all patients are customers or consumers, the field's enthusiasm and preparation for any new adaptation is not a given and remains a focus for empirical examination.

Focusing on the People Who Are Primary Care Physicians

The need for primary care to transform itself once again to maintain relevance in the twenty-first century American health system makes the primary care workforce a major sociological focus. For example, are younger PCPs better positioned to adapt to the medical-home model or other new external developments affecting their work than older colleagues? How do the value systems and expectations of younger PCPs, if different from older PCPs, shape what primary care work and the everyday experience look like, and what is possible in the future? These types of questions inform our ability to predict the trajectory of primary care as a set of careers. This trajectory will speak volumes about whether or not primary care work, for example, can meet the demands of a medical-home model by pulling back from increased routinization, faster pacing, ongoing skills erosion, and decreased autonomy on the part of PCPs. It will also help us predict the future prestige and place of primary care within the larger U.S. medical profession.

Younger physicians generally want a better lifestyle than their predecessors. More of them loathe thinking of medicine as a twenty-four-hour-a-day calling. Fewer take on the risks and rewards of owning their own practice, instead opting for salaried employment with regular hours, pay, and expectations. But their expectations and choices arguably align better with a primary care practice realm that treats its physicians less as independent professionals and more as labor inputs feeding into a production algorithm characterized by assembly-line medicine. If a new cohort of PCPs is to help save primary care, then it is important to know how their attitudes, behaviors, and experiences provide the grist for this salvation.

Greater numbers of women and international medical graduates (IMG) now fill primary care physician roles. Family medicine, pediatrics, and general internal medicine all substantially depend on these two groups for their future survival, since U.S.-born, white male medical students now have a keen aversion to becoming primary care physicians. It makes sense to better understand how these emerging groups think and act in their careers, and how they differ from their cohorts who have traditionally filled primary care jobs. Anecdotally, it is thought that significant numbers of young female physicians choose general primary care because they believe it offers the lifestyle flexibility favorable to building a family and raising children. From the IMG perspective, primary care careers offer the best and often only hope to gain entrance into the U.S. medical profession and to work as a physician in this country. This has raised questions about their commitment to primary care careers.[56] These particulars merit exploration of these new groups in primary care, in order to see how easily they align with medical-home particulars and the current demands of a transaction-focused primary care delivery system.

These two demographic groups also experience different challenges and opportunities compared to their white, U.S.-born male counterparts. For example, women professionals have been shown to earn less consistently than their male colleagues in the same job.[57] In primary care fields specifically, this has been found to be true.[58] Increasingly in medicine, women physicians have been shown to earn less than men even when fulfilling the same work roles and responsibilities.[59] But evidence that women physicians bring different qualities and talents to their jobs compared to men, qualities and talents that may foster the type of patient-centered care envisioned by the medical home, means that women PCPs factor as a major part of the human resource solution to reinvigorating primary care medicine in ways that move away from transactional, customer-focused medicine.

International medical graduates (IMGs), especially immigrant physicians, also will shape the future of primary care as a viable field of medicine. IMGs are constrained to begin their primary care careers in less desirable practice settings such as underserved rural and urban areas. They bring different expectations about salary and job responsibilities to their roles. In exchange for the opportunity to gain access to a prestigious occupation and to live here, immigrant physicians may accept lower pay, longer work hours, and more fragmented work responsibilities, at least early in their careers. They may encounter unique difficulties in their interactions with American patients due to language and communication barriers.

But because of where many IMGs are born, raised, and trained as physicians (outside of the United States and in resource-poor countries), they may appreciate how to interact with and deliver care to the uninsured patients in lower-cost ways that emphasize the ongoing honing of their decision-making skills through patient questioning, history taking, and the conduct of physical exams. These attributes, despite the language and communication barriers IMGs might face with some patients, can help achieve the ideal type of patient-centered care affiliated with the medical-home model: care that emphasizes the patient's voice and involves understanding the larger psychosocial contexts within which patients live and work.

Organization of the Book and the Physician Sample

This book is organized into two major sections. The first section describes the current everyday primary care work setting and how PCPs think and act within that setting. Through the eyes of PCPs, it tells the story of how primary care has changed over the past couple of decades and how PCPs have processed and adapted to the changes. A key point supported by these findings is that PCPs have acted strategically to align their thinking and behavior to the current business model in which they practice. The richness of the description offered in these chapters, combined with the attention paid to the PCP perspective, yields insights for fixing primary care and implementing the medical-home model discussed in the later chapters of the book.

The second section of the book explores the three demographic groups that are taking over primary care specialties: young physicians, women physicians, and IMGs. A sociological analysis is incomplete without considering how worker biographies shape individual responses to events in the surrounding external environment. For example, not everyone has the capacity or interest to adapt in the same manner to the changes imposed on them. These three demographic groups are the future of primary care, given the large percentage of primary care physicians over the age of fifty-five and the current large influx of both woman and IMGs into primary care.[60] Exploring their collective capacities to navigate the changes in primary care, as well as the unique perspectives each group offers, can help tell us more about how the primary care physician workforce will think and act in the future.

The PCPs interviewed for this book come from a variety of different demographic backgrounds and work settings. As a result, the findings are representative of contemporary primary care physicians and workplaces. PCPs from the three primary care specialties—family medicine, internal medicine, and pediatrics—are significantly represented in the sample. A variety of PCPs at different age and career stages are included, as well as large numbers of both males and females. Residents, students, medical leaders in primary care, medical educators, and, most importantly, the "in the trenches" practicing PCP all have a voice in this study. The appendix at the end of the book describes this sample and the study design in greater detail.

The vast majority of primary care delivery in the United States is still performed in smaller group practice settings but increasingly under the umbrella of a larger corporate entity that assumes the administrative and business roles for the groups. Many of the practicing PCPs participating in this study work in these types of settings. While other primary care delivery settings do exist, such as urgent care centers and retail clinics, most PCPs still work in traditional primary care offices. In addition, the study also includes PCPs practicing in academic and health center or clinic-type settings, where there are sicker and more indigent patients, but where an increasing number of primary care services are provided.

This book is a snapshot, not a longitudinal study. It does not include the patient viewpoint, which is a necessary and important compliment to the view of providers. These are valid limitations, and the findings must be considered in light of them. But as a snapshot it gives an accurate look at today's primary care world, both generally and through a provider-focused lens. As such, it informs those who wish to know more about what things look like and where they might be headed. It incorporates developments in primary care and the larger health care system of which it is a part to identify current challenges, lost opportunities, and future adaptations that interact to shape primary care work and physicians in the future.

To begin an analysis that focuses on the work and workers of primary care, it makes sense to address two fundamental questions: What does the typical primary care workday look like at present, and how has that workday evolved over time?

Part I

The Work of Primary Care

Chapter 2

A Typical Workday in Primary Care

During 2006, over 900 million medical care visits were made to doctors in the United States, with just over half made to family practitioners, internists, pediatricians, and OB/GYNs.[1] That's over three visits per year, per person. The typical PCP works between fifty and sixty hours per week, with the majority of that time spent in direct patient care.[2] That's ten to twelve hours a day, five days a week.

The typical primary care doctor in a recent national compensation survey earned just under $200,000 per year, compared to average salaries two and three times greater for certain surgical specialties, radiology, cardiology, and a variety of internal medicine subspecialties.[3] Salaries for primary care physicians have not kept pace with inflation, decreasing 10 percent after adjusting for inflation between 1995 and 2003.[4] Younger PCPs starting out often earn less—up to $50,000 to $60,000 less. Divide fifty-five hours per week (the average) into $190,000 and the hourly rate for a typical PCP is approximately $69 an hour. After taxes, that amounts to approximately $41 an hour. If a couple hundred thousand dollars in training debt are owed on the cost of a medical education, which is typical among a lot of younger PCPs, then this hourly rate decreases further. This rate does not qualify PCPs for food stamps, but it is clearly at the bottom in comparison to other medical specialties.

To maintain this salary, nothing else is as economically important for a primary care practice as ensuring an adequate number of billable office visits each day. For PCPs, it involves clearing away all other disturbances to focus on that objective, acting strategically to move through visits in a predictable manner, and delivering medicine that mixes large amounts of routine work in with sporadic and unpredictable doses of the nonroutine. Talking to PCPs, I found that their initial descriptions of the basic structure of the typical work-day were similar, regardless of whether they were family doctors, internists, or pediatricians.

> We schedule new patients for thirty minutes, established patients for fifteen. I'll see twenty to twenty-five patients per day. I generally try to work on a maximum of four patients an hour, and they get my full attention for fifteen minutes per patient and any follow-up. All our records are computer based, so my day can begin the moment I wake up. I will frequently log on to the system before going to the office, check and see if anything's come in overnight like lab results, check to see if there are any e-mails I have to address. I get to the office and start seeing patients about 9 A.M. each day, see patients continuously through 5 P.M., with an hour break for lunch. (Martin, family physician)

. . .

> I'm up out of bed about 6:30, and leave the house around 7:30. I usually have about half an hour for some paperwork, catch up on some things, and then my first office visit is scheduled for 8 A.M. I see patients from 8 A.M. to noon, usually take an hour for lunch. And during lunch I may make some patient calls, or do prescription refills, and then I try to eat something. Sometimes I run over a little bit. But I see patients from 1 until 5. The last one is scheduled for 4:30. Then I sit around and finish up paperwork, make some phone calls to patients, and I'm on the road by 6. If I'm not on call, then 50 percent of the time I take home some work. And we can do that because we have an electronic medical record, and we can do things like finish our charting at home, or creating new notes around labs I want done, etc. I probably put in another two hours at home each day, most of the time. The weeks we're on call, it's all by phone. We might get on a busy evening four or five calls, and you tell people "here's a refill for your medicine, or come see me tomorrow, or go to the emergency room if it's really serious." I'm seeing eighteen to twenty patients right now, but ideally it should be twenty-five or so. I'm still new and building my practice. (Lou, internist and pediatrician)

. . .

> We usually start seeing patients about eight or so, and go to about 4 or 4:15. That's the nice thing—it's pretty much Monday to Friday. We don't do any hospital medicine here. Probably see about twenty-five to thirty patients a day on average. There are a lot of forms for the patient, their insurance company, and we have people who do that but I might get

involved for getting preauthorizations for services or things like that. (Gary, internist)

. . .

We're all of the same mindset here, and that's to be able to finish everything by 5 or 5:15 so we can go home and enjoy our families. In the course of a day, I'll do between fifteen and twenty routine visits with kids, physicals or well-baby checkups for example, and have about ten to fifteen sick visits. That varies a bit by time of year. In the summer, there'll be fewer sick kids so I'll try and do more of the physicals since parents don't want kids to miss school for that kind of stuff. But in the winter, I have more illness coming through the practice. (Steven, pediatrician)

All of the interviewees talked about their day as one of seeing patients in batches of three or four per hour. Little time was spent during the "nine-to-five" part of the workday on leaving their office for anything, including lunch.

I usually try and grab something to eat around midday, and we'll not schedule patients for an hour or so to catch up and give the staff time for lunch. But, I often run late and will finish my morning patients during that time off, which leaves me only a half hour or so to get something to eat, return any urgent phone calls from patients, check labs and other stuff that might've come in, and get ready for my afternoon patients. There's really not much free time in my day to do anything else. (Tom, internist and pediatrician)

Seeing a targeted number of patients each day in the office to remain fiscally viable was emphasized more than any other aspect of the typical workday.

Patients don't understand. If I don't get them into the office, I don't get paid. It's that simple. They all want me to call them with this test result, or to answer a question they have that might keep them out of the office, but that's time I spend that has no reimbursement associated with it. For me or the practice. (Greg, internist and pediatrician)

In a business model that only pays for face-to-face visits, sick patients are needed so they can be brought into the office, seen, and a reimbursable bill can be generated. This redefines a "productive" PCP as one who can see many patients in a given day. The Center for Studying Health Systems Change reports that about three-quarters of all physicians (PCPs and specialists) in group practices have some part of their compensation tied to financial incentives.[5] In almost three-quarters of these cases, that compensation is dependent on physicians meeting individual productivity targets in their work, for example, the number of patients seen, number of procedures performed, and number of patients signed up in one's practice. In turn, almost three-quarters of physicians with compensation tied to productivity think the incentives themselves are important factors in determining how much they get paid.[6]

PCPs were not always paid in these ways. Like most doctors, they used to get paid according to their "usual and customary" charge. This meant that they were reimbursed for mostly what they billed, and as long as what they billed was not so different from what colleagues in their geographic area billed, they got what they asked for.

> The golden age of medicine was the golden age because many patients paid in cash, insurance companies paid you the rate you set, and there were only two insurance companies to deal with, Medicare and the Blues. It was clean, simple, there were relatively no hassles, and very little second guessing of what you did and how you did it. (Tony, internist)

But as specialty medicine grew, and many specialists like cardiologists began doing (and getting paid more for) things PCPs used to do, primary care reimbursements shrunk. Efforts were made in the 1990s to better compensate what PCPs did relative to their specialist counterparts. But these initial adjustments have not kept pace with the widening disparity between primary care and specialist reimbursement. In addition, reimbursement formulas also have not changed meaningfully to accommodate the time needed to treat what is unarguably a sicker population moving through primary care exam rooms on any given day. The emphasis on procedural over cognitive medicine is also a reality that makes much of the clinical work PCPs now do less profitable.

> You can't survive in an environment where Medicare pays you less today for the same thing than they did five years ago. It's not sustainable. So your only choice is to see more patients. (Rick, internist)
>
> . . .
>
> No one will pay you for time. They'll pay you to do a colonoscopy. They'll pay you to do a cardiac catheterization. They'll pay you to set a bone. They'll pay you to take out a cataract. But they're not going to pay you for time. (Rose, internist)
>
> . . .
>
> Our system pays for procedural medicine, not cognitive medicine. A dermatologist gets $400 for removing some lesion on a patient that takes an hour, and I have to fight to get $80 for an hour of talking with the patient about how to better take care of themselves. (Charlie, family physician)

In this type of reimbursement environment, it is in a primary care practice's best interest to move as many patients through its exam rooms as possible each day, because the costs of running the practice remain the same. This is why most PCP office settings go out of their way to turn no patient away, to "double book" their doctors to make sure there are enough patients to maintain adequate revenue, to limit interaction with patients through nonreimbursable phone calls and e-mail, and to incentivize physicians to keep visits as short as possible. In such a tightly packed, pressurized work environment, one glitch in a workday, one or two sicker-than-usual patients in the schedule, too many new patients, patients with complicated lab results, or too many patients who ask lots of questions once in the exam room can wreak havoc on a PCP's attempt to move through his or her day efficiently. Many PCPs in the study spoke of an apprehension they faced when walking into their exam rooms that the visit before them would turn into something more than a "cut-and-dried" diagnostic encounter.

> You never really know what you're going to get once you're in with the patient. They could be there for a headache, or sinus infection. But then once they get you in that room, they start to open up. And it usually happens for me right when I am about to put my hand on that doorknob to turn it and get out of there. They'll say, "Oh, just one more thing," or "Can I ask you about something else?" And I'll cringe sometimes because I don't know what's coming and I've got a couple other patients sitting in other rooms waiting to see me. (Wilma, family physician)
>
> .   .   .
>
> More than 50 percent of my practice now is kids who come in with some physical or surface complaint, like stomach pain or headaches, and the end result will be some behavioral issue that is the thing affecting them. As a pediatrician, you want to get at that. But it gets so you almost expect it in a certain number of encounters each day. It can take a long time, because we don't get trained to do that kind of stuff and you can go as deep as you want to go with the patients in a lot of the situations. It's a reality, but you know when you are seeing a lot of these situations in your day, everything's going to get backed up, you're going to run late, and you may be tempted to rush it in ways that aren't good for the patient. It's stressful on the families, and it's stressful on you. And so you can start out every day saying to yourself, "OK, what's going to pop up today and how do I intend to deal with it." (Leann, pediatrician)

PCPs in the study were fully aware of the reimbursement realities before them. Everyone understood that their pay was ultimately dependent on how many patients they could see in any given day, week, or year. When they talked about their days, they talked about the need to "make their numbers." It amazed me how accepting PCPs were when I asked them for the number of patients they saw in an average day. Instead of getting defensive or emphasizing that the numbers were not that important, they provided daily patient volume goals in a manner that was natural and accepted by them. Several of them spoke of patient visit expectations like a salesperson paid on commission might speak of the number of carpets they had to sell in a given day or week to earn a decent living.

PCPs did not express anger or frustration about how the need to generate visits affected their work. They fully accepted their workplace reality. As such, most spoke somewhat dispassionately about the issues raised for themselves and their interactions with patients by the assembly-line nature of their day.

In order to make ends meet around here, we need to see about twenty-eight patients a day. It's very difficult to see and deal with a patient in fewer than fifteen minutes, in a primary care setting, because you need to greet them, review all the information that's available, and one of the responsibilities of a primary care physician is to make sure that no stones are left unturned. Every time a patient comes into the office, it's an opportunity to make sure nothing's been missed by you or any other of the physicians who've been treating that person up to this point in time. So the diabetic patient may come in with a sore throat, but you feel like you can't just look at their sore throat and let them go. If you're doing your job right, you look at their entire diabetic treatment plan and make sure they haven't fallen behind on their A1c's,[7] on their lipids, on their foot exams, on their eye exams. If they're women, you want to take a quick look at their history and make sure that their mammograms have been done, that their GYN exams have been done. If they're coronary artery disease patients, you take a quick look and make sure they've had lipids done, and that they are on track. And you don't need to necessarily do anything at that visit, because you can't, but you need to make provisions to deal with it in some foreseeable period of time. That's what a primary care physician does. He or she ties all that stuff together. And that takes time. There is no way to do that in fewer than fifteen minutes and still have the time to interrelate with people. What you do give up, if you fall behind, is the opportunity to talk with people on a personal basis. (Mark, internist)

.   .   .

The constraints of time that are put upon us because of reimbursement issues demands that you move right through the visit and get where you need to go, cut out talking about their golf game and how the kid's high school graduation went because there isn't really time for that. And if you ask me how much time I should spend with a patient, I would say more is better. If I spent twenty minutes with a patient, I would've gotten more information and developed a better relationship with them than if I had spent fifteen. And you see doctors who really can't get it done because they're in there spending a half hour with every patient. You have to find a practice style that allows you to move efficiently and do the things you need to do and not turn the patient off, so they go, "Well, I'm not going to see that jerk again." (Charlie, family physician)

. . .

You've got to see a certain number of patients, it's that simple. So you learn ways of being more directive in that exam room, with the parents especially. Get them and you to focus on what is the most pressing issue they are in for, and try and be efficient in how you get them on the same page as you. Otherwise, you start falling behind and the day can become a nightmare. (Maura, pediatrician)

The Ironies of Shorter Patient Visits

The average length of an established patient office visit in primary care is around fifteen minutes.[8] This has remained steady during the first part of the twenty-first century. Primary care office visits are on average somewhat shorter than specialist office visits, which is ironic since doing primary care right, in theory, involves approaching patients holistically. By design, this takes more time because you have to ask about more things and consider them in their totality. It often means dealing with patients with multiple conditions that require extended history taking and counseling, and can involve vague presentations of symptoms and complaints that result in extended testing, communication, and decision making. In addition, PCPs experience more variety in terms of patients' presenting complaints and symptoms than, say, the average orthopedist who is setting fracture after fracture, or the average cardiac surgeon putting in stent after stent.

If someone comes in with a sore throat, a fifteen-minute visit is probably fine. For the majority of our patients, though, they have multiple medical problems. Especially if you have an established practice and you're treating an elderly or an adult population. The most common diagnoses are diabetes, hypertension, hyperlipidemia, and coronary disease. Those are the big four. And to address the issues that you need to for each one of those problems, at every visit, requires a half hour. But we don't always have a half hour for those patients. There are checklists of evaluations you have to do on each one of those patients and for each one of those diseases to make sure that they're adequately maintained and keeping up with the standards, and they're not progressing onto a worsening disease state. Specifically, for diabetes you can spend fifteen minutes just going over their diet and making sure they're checking their pulses and looking at the bottoms of their feet and whether or not they have numbness or tingling in their hands. All those are signs of progression of disease that are setting them up for a heart attack or stroke in the future. So we try to make sure we're staving those things off on a regular basis. If you said to me, "Well, what's the ideal number of patients?" I would say that depends. If they're all routine sick patients, quick sick visits, I would say thirty patients a day is doable. If you had diabetes, hypertension, or hyperlipidemia with every patient you saw, you probably couldn't see more than sixteen patients a day. (Francis, family physician)

The fifteen-minute visit is the normative standard for the basic, acute care visit in primary care. To see how ingrained its acceptance was in the PCP psyche, all I had to do was listen to how several of the doctors in the study spoke about visits that might extend to twenty minutes or longer. For some, twenty-minute visits were an unachievable luxury, coveted and capable of achieving higher-quality medicine. It seemed far-fetched that another five minutes with a patient could produce such differences in the quality of care. Others spoke defiantly of their own decisions to forfeit income in order to have longer visits with their patients, as if their choice to spend an extra five or ten minutes in the exam room was akin to making a significant personal sacrifice.

I kind have made a compromise income-wise by only seeing twenty to twenty-five patients a day. My income's probably at the bottom compared to my internal medicine partners. But it allows me to have a different kind of relationship with my patients. I try not to rush them in and out, and stay on time, and people appreciate that. (Sal, internist)

. . .

In this practice, we don't worry so much about seeing enough patients to make a certain amount of money. Maybe that's not smart on our part. But we feel we are doing this more than just for the money, and that as long as we all feel our compensation is adequate, we can do fewer visits and get more of the other things from the job we want. (Leann, pediatrician)

Shorter visits have forced PCPs to become more standardized and strategic in how they conduct patient encounters. Many PCPs interviewed spoke of an imperative in every visit to direct patient interaction from beginning to end if they were to avoid falling behind in the workday. Harry, a young internist, gave a sense of this approach in describing visits with chronic-disease patients:

The staff will check out the patient beforehand, check their vitals and see if they need any prescription refills. They write a very little brief reason for the visit at the top of the note, which is helpful because then you know what you are going in for. I'll review my last note on the patient, skim the chart, and check any notes that might have come in from specialists between the current visit and the patient's last previous visit with me. To see if there is anything extra we need to talk about. And usually I've written down something at the last visit that says, "OK, the next time the patient comes in make sure to talk about X, Y, and Z." That refreshes my memory. I walk into the room, say why I think the reason is for their visit, ask them if they have any particular issues they would like to discuss, and if they don't, I pretty quickly go more into what I think the reason for the visit is. For instance, if it's diabetes, OK, how are your finger sticks looking, are you checking your feet every day, are you seeing an eye doctor once a year, how are you tolerating the medications, are you exercising enough?

I go through a brief review of systems, ask them if they have any chest pains or shortness of breath or bowel or bladder problems. Anything like that. Move through the physical. And then at the end of a quick physical exam that's tailored to what their medical issues are, discuss what the plan is, whether any changes need to be made in medications, what the next steps for follow-up will be, referrals if necessary. I try to approach it the same way with every patient because I find it helps me to flow more smoothly, so if I deal with every patient in a similar way, I can stay on track with the time allotted for visits. (Harry, internist)

There are advantages to PCPs becoming more directed and efficient in the conduct of a patient visit. It allows different patients to become the beneficiaries of standard interactions with the physician, which guarantees a minimum level of quality care. It also lets the doctor who is the knowledge-expert guide the discussion, and facilitates the recognition and treatment of a patient's chief complaint quickly in some instances. However, an implicit danger for patient care arises in PCPs' psychological adjustment to shorter visits and higher workloads. This danger is the potential to miss something important that might underlie the patient's chief somatic complaint or that is not initially part of the complaint at all. It could also produce dissatisfied patients. As we will see in Chapter 5, a significant part of the nonroutine aspect of PCP's work involved playing detective during a visit and probing through a conversation, listening whether or not there were other diagnoses or medical issues harder to see yet still affecting the patient. The chief threats in this regard were the existence of clinical diagnoses related to depression or other mental health issues.

> In primary care, it's unpredictable. You go to the orthopedist with a sore shoulder, and that's where it stops. You go to the primary care doctor because you have a stomach ache and it winds up that you're depressed, and you're an alcoholic, and your husband's just died. And all this other stuff crops up, which is the kind of stuff that you can't simply delay until the next visit. You've got to sometimes really work with the patient to get this stuff out. Or sometimes you don't, it comes out quick but then you've got to engage the patient more to figure it out.
>
> And the fifteen-minute visit has now become the forty-minute visit, and now you're behind. So, you never really know what's behind the door. And 60 percent of the time it ends up being some social issue that you need to give the time to, give the person some direction and support because they're not going to feel better unless their life situation is better. You need to be able to negotiate that, sense that, and simply not throw medicine blindly at a problem that medicine won't be able to cure. (Mark, internist)
>
> .   .   .
>
> You never know when you might get blindsided by a patient you've never seen before. Or people that say they have one problem, but then you get them in the room and it's a whole other can of worms. You do your best to listen to as much as possible. (Wilma, family physician)
>
> .   .   .
>
> The two biggest complaints we get here in this practice are fatigue and insomnia. Very nonspecific. And when you start to delve into it, to try and get a better idea of what they are talking about, a lot of it winds up being social problems. A lot of people expect to be able to take a pill to make them feel better. We see more and more patients come in with these complaints. Antidepressants are in my top five most prescribed drugs now, whereas they weren't fifteen years ago. But to get at the

underlying real problem, it takes time. I have to go through a bunch of different things the symptoms could be reflective of, I have to sometimes order blood work and tests, and then, if nothing is turning up, I broach with the patient that this could be reflective of something more like depression. And there's no blood test I can do for depression. There's no approach to diagnosing it that doesn't take some time and individualized approach to the patient. In the end, it's really about listening to the patient, and ruling out other diagnoses. But it's a real diagnosis. (Mick, family physician)

An irony-in-the-making existed each workday for PCPs. To excel within the business model in which they now found themselves, and to be considered "good" doctors that could navigate a full patient load efficiently, they needed to develop personal styles and work behaviors that allowed them greater speed without sacrificing their ability to get the primary patient diagnosis right. However, in taking this approach, they lessened their ability to uncover secondary problems affecting patients, problems that after the visit might grow into real illnesses for patients. Being a good PCP in the early twenty-first century at times sounded more like being akin to an army medic—address the core clinical issue, get it right, patch it up, and move the patient out. It meant executing several paradoxical work styles simultaneously—fast yet deliberate, standardized yet idiosyncratic, and verbose yet silent. It required PCPs who could think on their feet, exhibit flexibility, and not let perfection become the enemy of good care provision.

Teams, Nonphysician Providers, and Their Role in the Typical PCP Workday

Much is made about the potential provided by the use of a clinical team approach and nonphysician providers to alleviate primary care physician workloads and improve the efficiency of primary care medical delivery. Teams can reduce medical errors, increase work productivity, and deliver higher-quality patient care.[9] Within the medical-home approach proposed as a means to revitalize primary care, the team-based practice model looms as a central facilitator in providing patient-centered care.[10] This approach would use nurse practitioners and physician assistants in a partnership role with PCPs, who would retain overall authority over care management and coordination in the practice. It would also make registered nurses, traditionally the assistants of PCPs, more involved in certain aspects of clinical care. The clinical team approach now used in primary care ranges from physicians and nurses interacting in an ad hoc manner around individual patient visits to formal protocols and procedures used in primary care practices that give greater independence in the delivery of patient care to nurse practitioners (NPs) and physicians' assistants (PAs).

Almost all of the PCP practices in the study used NPs and PAs extensively as substitute labor, meaning that these nonphysician clinicians took the place of PCPs in lower-complexity care situations for the main purpose of generating greater profit for the practice. They earned much less than PCPs, yet insurance reimbursements for their work was on a par with what PCPs received. As a result, this labor was not used in a team-based approach to patient care, as suggested by the medical-home model, where the same patient benefited from a group clinical effort with different individuals who provided unique expertise. Instead, PCPs used NPs and PAs as lower-priced clinicians who could see, on their own, a percentage of the routine care flowing through the office on a given day. That is, the most common use of these "physician extenders" by PCPs was in giving them their own patient visit schedules, getting them also to focus on generating visit volume and basic acute care, and not using them in integrated, innovative ways to deliver greater patient-centered care.

> We have more of the nurse practitioners here than we had a few years ago. They see a lot of the acute care, simple stuff, and that frees me up to do the complex things. I see very little of the simple stuff anymore, the head colds, ear aches. That's all seen by midlevel providers in the office. Because I have to delegate my time where it's best used. (Rick, internist)
>
> . . .
>
> I can hire a PA now and they'll get 85 percent of what I get for the same visit. I can pay them a decent wage and still make money off what they do. So I now oversee four different offices, and employ mainly NPs and PAs in them. They are good, they know what they're doing, and then I can play the role of consultant if they run into a problem. Otherwise, they work on their own. Completely independent. That leaves my schedule to focus only on the more severe or nonroutine cases, and so I move around from office to office seeing those patients while my physician extenders take care of most of the rest. (Bill, internist)
>
> . . .
>
> Let's admit it. We use more NPs and PAs because it's cheaper for us. That's it. That's the reality. And if it wasn't cheaper, we wouldn't use them as much. But it's not to enhance quality. There are very good NPs and PAs, don't get me wrong. But the training of a physician, four years of medical school, residency, all the boards you have to take—that doesn't compare to the training of an NP or PA. (Matt, family physician)

Internal-medicine practices participating in the study appeared to use NPs and PAs the most in their daily work, with pediatricians employing them to a much lesser extent. The typical arrangement involved a ratio of perhaps one non-physician clinician for every two or three PCPs in a given practice. It was clear from discussions with PCPs that they viewed these individuals as providers in their own right, more limited in their scope of work than themselves, yet able to function independently to provide a chunk of the practice's care. They did not refer to them as "team members" but instead as practitioners answerable for their own productivity and ability to see a certain number of patients each day.

With respect to the presence of registered nurses who worked directly with PCPs, it appeared that PCPs relied on them mostly for less complex work that facilitated a quicker patient visit. This was true regardless of the PCP's gender. These nurses provided a host of services around the actual exam room encounter between PCP and patient. They typically obtained patient vital signs (weight, blood pressure), recorded the patient's chief complaint for the physician, helped execute physician orders such as lab testing and radiologic exams, assisted with referrals to specialists, followed up with patients on test results, arranged subsequent patient appointments with a specialist, and conveyed PCP orders on follow-up care to patients. Many PCPs spoke with fervor about the facilitating role played by their nurses in helping them move through a busy workday. For many of them, competent nurses assisting them were more valuable than any other asset and more important than an electronic medical record or standardized clinical guideline. They were key members of the "physician team," but their team role was segmented and confined to doing the scut work of patient preparation for the physician encounter.

> My nurse is worth her weight in gold. I'm telling you, without her help, forget about it. And we've worked together a long time, so she knows how I like to do things, and I can trust her to take care of as much as possible around my actual time with the patient. (Brad, internist)
>
> · · ·
>
> Have you met any of the nursing staff here? Well, they're tremendous. They keep me moving through my visits, they'll find a way to get hold of me if I'm spending too long with a patient, try and find ways to speed me up if I'm behind. Especially when someone with diabetes or hypertension comes in. They'll pull the patient's info, see what's due to be done, if it's an exam or a meds check or whatever, put that into the electronic note for me to see before I walk into the room, and they're doing this while I'm still in the room with another patient. (Lou, internist and pediatrician)

What the Typical Workday Does to PCPs and Primary Care

The typical PCP workday is a hectic, office-based, eight-to-ten-hour affair built on the need for speed in moving through patient visits while still providing good care. There are dangers in this reality. First, there is clear evidence in health care and other industries of the inverse link between the speed and quality of production. Doing more of something may make you better at it, but doing more of it too quickly raises the possibility of things being overlooked, and of more mistakes occurring. Would we feel confident if our automobile mechanics built no cushion into their workday to deal with unexpected or uncertain situations that inevitably arise in the course of fixing automobiles? More to the point, how does the emphasis on a fast-paced production model make the worker feel? Does any job remain as intellectually gratifying and satisfying when the primary pressure is to do it quicker? One of the dangers in focusing any worker, skilled or unskilled, primarily on production is that it undermines the ability of that worker to derive meaning from the work he or she does. This meaning stems from feeling control over the work itself, over the decisions that get made in doing the work, and from an ingrained sense that what one is doing is important, requiring the worker and no one else for it to be completed successfully.

This raises another point that speaks to the effects of a volume-driven business model on the prestige of primary care. If substitute labor, less intensely trained and lower paid, must be used in purely instrumental ways by PCPs hoping to "fill production gaps" in their everyday practice, where does that dynamic find its logical end? Twenty years ago, few primary care physicians likely thought that any portion of their work was easily "substitutable" using lower-skilled labor. Now, the pressures of production have forced an acknowledgment by PCPs that NPs and PAs can do a fair number of routine things in primary care, and that using them produces more profit for the practice as a whole.

But as the pressure to see more patients continues in primary care, will that acknowledgment be broadened to include previously "too complex" areas of primary care medicine? If so, how would we begin to look at primary care?

In the short-term solution of using cheaper, less-skilled labor to meet production demand, the field of primary care risks its image as something only MDs and their traditional primary care practices can do best. This may empower new delivery structures such as retail clinics and urgent care centers that employ greater numbers of nonphysician clinicians to do more types of primary care medicine in the future. For a medical field already suffering from image problems–from medical students, other specialists, and some in the general public–this tactical misstep can render a larger strategy to assert greater control over the primary care work domain less effective.

Chapter 3

How the Primary Care Workday Has Changed

How has the typical PCP workday changed over time, besides the obvious emphasis on volume and shorter visits? Table 1 presents other meaningful aspects of the evolution of the PCP workday, identified through the study data. According to older PCPs, the most profound clinical change is that chronic-disease patients make up an increasingly larger proportion of an internist's or family doctor's workday. The fraction of the patient population with one or more chronic diseases ranged from half to three-quarters among PCPs in the study.

> The typical conditions I see are acute things, like upper respiratory infections and bronchitis. I see a lot of chronic conditions. I would say a third to half of my day is spent just with patients who are diabetic or are prediabetic. Hypertension and hyperlipidemia also make up another good chunk of my patient population on a given day. (Martin, family physician)

The typical internist or family physician was affected by trends in the aging population and rising rates of chronic diseases such as hypertension, diabetes, and depression. Sicker patients now appeared in the PCP's office compared to ten or twenty years ago. This was especially true for many mid- and late-career PCPs with established patient populations who had grown older with their doctors. Half of U.S. citizens have a chronic disease, and half of those have two or more chronic diseases. The most prevalent chronic diseases involve hypertension, heart disease, mental health disorders, and diabetes.[1] Almost 40 percent of Medicare-eligible individuals have three or more chronic conditions.[2]

Table 1 Comparing the Workday of a PCP Now and 30 Years Ago

Criterion	Then	Now
Workday hours	6 or 7 A.M. to 5 or 6 P.M., more if needed at hospital later in day	8 or 9 A.M. to 5 or 6 P.M., more if accessing electronic medical record systems off-site
Chief workday disturbances	Hospital admission or emerging issue with hospital patient	Insurance-related issues (e.g., preauthorizations) and doing patient call-backs
Variety of work settings	Hospital, office, irregular out-of-office networking opportunities with peers (meetings, etc.)	Office only, few out-of-office networking opportunities with peers
Call schedules	Frequent, daily or every few days	Infrequent, every few days, weeks, or weekends
Oversight of work	Little external oversight, professional standards maintained by PCP individually	Oversight through performance monitoring, and use of standardized clinical guidelines that structure PCP work in many areas
Type of work performed in office	Mostly cognitive medicine, some procedures, some insurance-related patient advocacy work, some coordination of specialist care	Almost all cognitive medicine, regular and increasing insurance-related patient advocacy work, high degree of coordination of specialist care; heavy chronic disease and behavioral health management
Out-of-visit patient contact	Less expected and less performed	Expected and performed daily by PCPs or their nurses
Patient expectations	Lower, accepting of delays and going back for information	Higher, expect quicker turnarounds
Health of patient population	Chronic disease but lower incidence and less complex clinical management expectations, healthier younger adults and children, fewer elderly	Sicker populations throughout the life span, complex management expectations for chronic diseases, more elderly, more children and adults with psychosocial issues
Types of patients	Fewer elderly, older chronic-disease populations	More elderly, large chronic-disease populations, large at-risk populations, including youth and adolescents

Table 1   Continued

Criterion	Then	Now
Fiscal reality	Take time with patients, try and do as many things as provider competence and patient needs allow, including procedures—get paid for them; being jack-of all-trades is key strategic goal of provider—keep patient from specialist if you can manage it	Every patient seen quickly is additional revenue earned; limiting time with patients key strategic goal of provider—know when it's time to refer patient to specialist, even if you think you can manage it, and refer quickly
Competition for the PC dollar	Little competition, specialists depend on PCP for referrals	Heavy competition—allied health professionals (NPs and PAs); urgent-care centers and retail medicine; subspecialists who claim to better manage niche conditions such as hypertension

Source: Summary derived from analysis of PCP interviews.

Our bread and butter are diabetes, hypertension, and high cholesterol. A lot of patients with one or more of these things. And these patients can be simpler to treat in a visit or more complex. You just don't know until they walk in. And the conditions are not simple to manage. I'm not a diabetic educator per se. But to manage diabetics correctly, I have to educate them about low blood sugar, about taking their medications on time, about medication interactions, the importance of exercise, etc. That takes some time. (Mick, family physician)

For general pediatricians, the biggest change compared to ten or twenty years ago is the increased number of children experiencing behavioral health issues, ranging from mild bouts of anxiety to more serious instances of depression and bipolar disorder. Pediatricians in the study speculated on average that a quarter to one-half of their total pediatric patient visits dealt with some behavioral health issue. Part of the reason their offices had become the epicenter for identification and diagnosis of childhood behavioral health issues was the shortage of child psychiatrists and psychologists in almost every community, creating long waits for visits and treatment. Another reason was that many children remained undiagnosed for behavioral disorders until they presented in a primary care setting for another symptom or clinical problem.

Compounding the problem of sicker, more complex patients was a second change in primary care work: the increasing use of clinical guidelines and other quality improvement mechanisms that standardized patient care but increased the PCP's administrative and clinical demands during a given visit.[3] In the age of evidence-based medicine, good disease prevention and management translates into higher-quality care for the patient, but it also produces a more compact, varied workload for the PCP compared to the past. Charlie, a longtime family physician, discussed the paradox of standardized disease prevention and management:

> It used to be when you came in and you had a cold, I took care of your cold and that was it. Maybe I said I haven't seen you for five years and you need a check-up or a blood test. Now, when a patient comes in for their cold, we have a detailed problem list for each patient, and if you're doing your job right you won't just take care of the cold, you'll glance and see when they had their mammogram last, have they had a colonoscopy, when did they have their last physical, have they had their lipids checked recently, if there's any other risk factors showing up. That takes up a lot of time. The other thing that is very different is the management of any individual disease process in primary care. It's far different than it was twenty-five years ago.
>
> The best example is diabetes. We're clearly doing much better caring for diabetics now. Diabetes has serious complications. It used to be when you saw a diabetic in the office, you looked at all the individual blood sugar tests they had and you'd decide whether they need to change their medicine around. We never had to worry about diabetics' lipids, for example. And now, almost every diabetic is being managed with a medication like Lipitor. Because it's been shown that if you control a diabetics' lipids and blood pressure and sugars, they live longer and have fewer complications. We're supposed to monitor the urine tests, supposed to monitor the blood test, the lipids, the A1C, and examining the patient's foot and documenting that you looked for nephropathy. We're monitoring many things on a diabetic which we never did before, a lot of which involves a blood draw or exam. Every time you draw blood, there'll be a phone call to check that result and give it to the patient. Things are very different in the day-to-day management of a patient with chronic illness.
>
> So, when you see a patient in the office, instead of just treating the acute illness, you've got to get involved in the overall management of the patient and it can be pretty intense. Better care for the patient, of course, but it takes more time for the doctor. (Charlie, family physician)

Part of the problem is that the standards of care for both preventive and disease management activities in the twenty-first century are tomes that reflect precise knowledge of disease processes but little understanding of the typical PCP workday and its realities of high patient volume to make ends meet. Guideline complexity has been found to be a factor undermining primary care physician use and perception of clinical guidelines.[4] For example, the executive summary published by the American Diabetes Association (ADA) describing its 2007 standards of medical care for diabetes runs almost seven pages of single-spaced, full-page print and includes numerous diagnostic, treatment, and prevention-oriented activities in which the PCP should be involved.[5] Imagine the guidelines and standards of care in play when a patient with diabetes, obesity, hypertension, and depression presents for a fifteen-minute visit with a PCP. It is impossible for the PCP to provide "quality care" in compliance with one or multiple guidelines within a compressed time period. In addition, the physician-patient relationship suffers because PCPs get preoccupied with moving through a checklist rather than taking an updated history from their patients and communicating with them about their everyday lives. The chronic-disease visit becomes a standard transaction completed the same way for everyone.

PCPs who were interviewed talked about the negative by-products associated with standardizing aspects of their work such as chronic disease management. For example, being asked by an insurer to make sure, above all else, that patients have a hemoglobin A1C level of no more than 7 percent can shape how PCPs interact with each diabetic who comes into their exam rooms. On the plus side, it provides an easy clinical target for the PCPs to focus upon that is consonant with their felt pressures to keep visits short and move efficiently through the workday. But this psychological dynamic could affect care on an individual patient basis in ways that cause dissatisfaction on the part of both the physician and the patient.[6]

> Every patient is different. You can't just take some guideline and use it and assume that you got everything on the patient, or that the patient's happy because you checked their blood levels or did some thing on a checklist. Patients want you to listen to them. And most of them want you to explain what you're looking at and why. (Hannah, family physician)
>
> .   .   .
>
> Knowing I don't have a lot of time, and I have to document all these things I did for a patient with hypertension or diabetes, I can't go into that room and get into a lot of chit-chat. The things I used to like to do. I've got to focus and go through the different things I'm required to do.

And I'm not sure the patient even gets it. I don't know a lot of the time if they feel better that I have all these things I'm doing or if they feel like I'm just treating them like a widget. (Sam, family physician)

In the twenty-first century PCP office, clinical care guidelines turn into formal performance measures, which become the main way in which PCPs and their businesses are evaluated by those that pay them, the private insurers and government. This also creates additional dynamics not good for patient care. For example, PCPs may begin to see each patient as a contributor to a collective performance outcome rather than as an individual who might require unique understanding and approaches. PCPs may feel compelled to gravitate more toward "easier" patients, ones whose care standard can be met more quickly and with less work on the part of the PCP.

In fact, there is evidence of this "cherry picking" process in health care delivery.[7] This threatens to marginalize "noncompliant" and sicker patients for whom the applicable clinical standards of care are too voluminous to comply with in the timespan of basic office encounters. In a workday where high numbers of fifteen-minute appointments earn the most revenue, how many diabetics or hypertensive patients, or ones with both conditions, might a PCP want to see when a certain percentage of each will be of the noncompliant or sicker variety?

Ceding Control to the Corporation and Empowered Patients

A second change, forced onto PCPs both by the economics of primary care and the trend toward increased monitoring of their work, is that more are now salaried employees or quasi-owners working within larger primary care office networks or practices, instead of being full owners, perhaps with a few other PCPs, of a smaller practice. This evolution, traditionally referred to by sociologists as the "corporatization" of medical work, has been necessitated for several reasons: having "strength in numbers" when negotiating reimbursement rates with insurance companies; needing to distribute increasingly expensive practice overhead costs among a larger group of physicians; having an administrative apparatus that can efficiently manage the vast paperwork; and meeting technological demands now placed on PCPs. A recent national survey found that over one-third of PCPs said they either would not be able to support their practice overhead over the next five years, or they were doubtful they could.[8]

Much of the modern-day health-care-quality movement forces individual PCPs to give up direct involvement in the business side of medicine and hand it over to an umbrella corporation that can handle its expense and bureaucracy. Charlie is a family practitioner in his late fifties. He has been in practice for thirty years. He used to be part owner of a large primary care group practice. As the economics of medicine got tougher in the 1990s, his practice was sold to a large primary care network. Now Charlie is both a salaried employee and company shareholder. He has shares in the network company of which his practice is a part, which he has paid for, but he draws an annual salary from the company that can vary sporadically in the event his particular practice location, which consists of ten other PCPs, does poorly financially. And financial performance is measured strictly by the number of patients moving into and out of the office each day.

Like Charlie, more PCPs than ever before straddle an employment netherworld between independent business owners who get to make all the decisions and reap all the rewards, and paid employees who are subservient to a higher master who shields them from the risks of a competitive marketplace. For Charlie and some older PCPs who had practiced independently during that "golden age" of medicine referred to earlier, when doctors could name their price, this new practice model makes them work harder while being paid less:

> I made more ten years ago than I make now. And I was able to spend more time with my patients. Today, I have to see more patients just to try and get close to the income I was pulling down in the past. That's discouraging. (Charlie, family physician)
>
> .   .   .
>
> Interestingly enough, my salary has gone down every year over the past decade and yet I'm seeing substantially more patients. (Quentin, family physician)

But the positives of being a salaried employee in a larger organization outweighed the negatives for almost all PCPs. Older PCPs especially recalled the strategic reasons they had sought out larger group-practice models within which to do their jobs. Most of these reasons centered on the ongoing struggle between insurance companies and themselves, a struggle in which insurers were viewed as the enemy, cutting reimbursements at every corner, and forcing PCPs to work in unsatisfying ways. Steven, a pediatrician, told the story of how his group of a few pediatricians had moved itself in the 1990s toward becoming part of a large, multispecialty primary care practice, which ceded administrative control to a corporate structure that could fight the insurance companies for them.

> This practice consists of what used to be all smaller groups, what we call the cottage industry, and single docs. And we all had the fear of God put into us by a very large insurer when they were coming into the area,

because we had heard the horror stories of what they had done in other places. They would come in, offer you the world, get you on board, and then they would start cranking down the reimbursement to the point where they controlled the patient lives, and if you weren't willing to work for pennies on the dollar, then you weren't going to work at all. As they started to make waves about coming into the area, we picked physician groups that we were comfortable working with, and we banded together and spent more than a year trying to iron out how we were going to do this as a big group. And there was a group of internists doing the same thing, and a group of family docs, and so we all got together, and created this conglomerate. But it took a year of sitting down and putting it all together.

It was a lot of work. In the long run, it made our little group of docs here a much better practice. It puts us in a situation where we can make more demands of insurance companies where we couldn't before. As a small group, they'd say go ahead and leave. But when you have a group of seventy-five-plus providers, caring for hundreds of thousands of lives, now they have to sit up and take notice. We have more clout, as it were. As for giving up some of the autonomy to make our own decisions to the larger organization, well that's part of it. And then trying to get this large group of cottage industry docs to work together, it's been a struggle. The first two to five years were pretty tough, but it's gotten better as time goes on. The big thing that always causes conflict here and there is what the central business office wants versus what we in our own little practice think we want. (Steven, pediatrician)

Despite ceding administrative control, most of the PCPs belonging to these larger groups felt that they still had adequate autonomy over their local practices.

The people who founded this organization never wanted to micromanage us. They wanted us to practice the way we wanted to. And we have a lot of control here. We decide how much time we want to take off, how much we want to work, we have control over the kind of staff we want, and who those people will be. They help us with these things, but we get to make the final decisions. (Peggy, pediatrician)

These larger, corporatized environments take many of the business responsibilities for running a practice out of the PCP's hands. They allow fewer financial risks for individual PCPs who become responsible for a smaller share of the fixed overhead costs of the practice, rather than assuming the majority or all of the costs. In the opinions of many PCPs, they allow doctors to be doctors.

> I joined this practice nine years ago, and I've been happy here. The corporation handles the entire business side of things. The billing, dealing with the insurance companies, credentialing issues, dealing with staff and payroll. And you're basically allowed to practice medicine. You're salaried, but your salary is dependent on what you're bringing into the practice, and I like that end of it. So you can work as much or little as you want, and get paid accordingly. The corporation takes a percentage of your billings as overhead, administrative costs, and it's a pretty reasonable amount. And they make money off of us because they do our labs, our radiology stuff, because they have separate business entities in-house that do those things. They don't like to micromanage us. We can do pretty much what we want in our practice. But if we need help, they're there. It's kind of a symbiotic relationship. (Greg, internist and pediatrician)

> . . .

> I looked into borrowing the money to start my own practice. I went to banks, got all the details. And it would've been something like $800,000, which would've been a huge risk for something I thought would work well, but couldn't be sure. By joining this group, they allowed me to set up a line of credit with them, and then they paid for all the renovation of my office, getting it ready to go. Going with this group I get all the feedback I need on where the expenses are at, they help me draw a budget up each year, they advise me on personnel and supply costs, and it's like having wonderful central office that can take care of things. I don't have to spend my nights worrying about payroll or FICA taxes. It's a wonderful compromise. (Theresa, family physician)

Most importantly for some PCPs, joining corporate practice organizations created an everyday work environment where there were fewer personal responsibilities to be on call or available around the clock for patients. To PCPs who put lifestyle at the top of their priority list, which were the large majority of the younger and middle-age PCPs in the study, this type of employment setting was the only viable option for them. They saw owning their own practice as highly risky, impractical, and in direct opposition to their ability to emphasize their nonwork lives.

When I talked with Charlie about the changes that had occurred in his workday, it was seven in the morning. He was letting me interview him before his typical day of seeing patients started at eight o'clock. Charlie was frank about another change that has taken place in his day over the past ten or fifteen years. This change was the increased expectations of patients, and of how these expectations created greater complexity in a workday now defined by the constant pressure to produce high numbers of office visits.

> The workday that I do now has changed quite dramatically in twenty-five years. The computerization of medicine and the fax machine, everybody wants to know everything now. People come in and you see them and they need two tests, an X-ray and a blood test, and they want to know before the end of the afternoon what the answers were. It used to be that I would see my patients during the day and then I would get the lab work back in five to seven days and contact those that I needed to talk to about it. Whereas now I get it back the same day. I would guess now that for every hour we see a patient, we're probably doing fifteen to twenty minutes of work with lab data, X-ray data, calling the patient, calling the family. This adds 25 percent to your day. Which never used to happen. You used to see the patient, gather all the data, and then they'd come back and see you in ten days, and you'd say, "Well, this is where we are and this is what we need to do in the next step." But now everything is so instant that it almost can be overwhelming at times. That's the biggest change. (Charlie, family physician)

The desire for quicker service was cited by almost all PCPs as a major issue creating strain between themselves and patients, particularly during a workday where they had to schedule patients tightly in order to make ends meet. Pediatricians were especially vocal about the service demands placed on them by today's parents.

> The younger parents, they have big expectations. I think that it's part of their whole value system, of their generation and what they expect from everything. It's all about immediate gratification. When they want their kids to be seen, you have to see them right away, or they'll fly off to some urgent care center where the care will be less than ideal most of the time. Do they always need to bring their children in? Absolutely not. But if you try and use a nurse to triage them, to explain why they don't need to bring their child in, they'll just go somewhere else. They want you to see their child, tell them that everything is fine, and fix whatever it is that needs to be fixed with a pill or something fast. I think it stems more from what they get out of it. They want to feel like they're good parents.

Like they're doing the right thing always for their child. But it creates expectations and demands that are simply unrealistic. (Maura, pediatrician)

Most of the empathy expressed when interviewing PCPs about the service issue was directed at themselves and not their patients. In most of their discussions, PCPs were less tolerant or aware of the benefits for patients of having PCPs meet their expectations, particularly when it came to simpler things like communicating with patients outside of the office visit and in quicker ways. Some PCPs implied that expectations such as being seen on time or talking to patients by phone when they had a question were unreasonable, in large part because of the existing structure of their workday and the need to see a lot of patients. This attitude fed into a more paternalistic, negative view of patients.

People have no tolerance for waiting anymore. That's one of the biggest stresses. People just have no tolerance for anything other than themselves. So, for example, I was here last Monday and I had a patient who had an acute MI [myocardial infarction], a heart attack, and he went out in an ambulance, and then the next girl came in, and she ended up having meningitis, and so now I am way behind because those two came in as fifteen-minute follow-up visits, because the guy's presenting complaint was indigestion and earache, and the girl was put into the schedule as a headache, and they both wound up having serious things. Both of these people get wheeled out of here on stretchers, and the next patient in says, "Why are you running behind?" And I'm like, "Did you see what just went out through the waiting room?! Didn't you have to pick up your feet for the stretchers to go by you?!" And they're like, "Well, you're thirty minutes behind today." No tolerance for anything. People are so demanding. Not at all compassionate for their other human entities. (Rick, internist)

.   .   .

I run behind a lot. Because we have to schedule patients in fifteen-minute slots but if I feel I want to take longer, I do it. That backs me up almost every workday. And some patients have no tolerance for that. They want to be seen exactly when they're supposed to be seen. But, if they're my established patients, if they've been with me for awhile, then they know that if patients before them need me for longer, that I would do the same for them if they needed it. I would spend more time with them and someone else would have to wait longer. (Frank, internist)

Belief on the part of PCPs that patients want quicker service was coupled with their observations that increasing numbers of patients came to the office visit already armed with lots of speculative information related to what they thought was wrong with them. For PCPs, this complicated their job before they even walked into the exam room. As Charlie relayed from his own experiences:

> I had a patient walk in here recently and say to me that they thought they had myasthenia gravis. Now myasthenia gravis is a rare and unusual condition that I have probably seen in thirty-five years of practice four times. And I asked them, "What makes you think you have that?" He went through the symptoms, and the long and the short of it, once he went through the testing, that's what the patient had. That sort of thing never used to happen before. But at the same time patients come in and they've got a little bit of GI upset and a little bit of bloating, and it may just be stress, but they now come in and say, "I'm sure I have ovarian cancer and I need to have a pelvic CT scan and I need a CA-125 blood test and a pelvic ultrasound because I read on the Internet that if you think you have these symptoms you have to go to the doctor and get checked for ovarian cancer." And with all due respect, there have been all sorts of great studies done on whether it's cost-effective to do routine screening for ovarian cancer. And the answer is no. And you get families that come in and say, "Aunt Sally had ovarian cancer. I want to get an ultrasound and a blood test." The art of medicine is deciding which one of those patients you'll never see again if you don't order the tests, so you order them. Or which one can you convince that maybe it's not the most necessary thing since they don't have any symptoms at all, or ones that could be a million other things more likely. (Charlie, family physician)

Many people now use the Internet to try and get information on their symptoms. The Pew Internet and American Life Project found that eight in ten Internet users search for health information online, with two-thirds of these users searching for information on a specific disease or medical problem, and over half to gain information on a medical treatment or procedure.[9] In addition, Pew also reported that 85 percent of women and 75 percent of men surveyed had searched for health information at least once in the past.[10] The Pew surveys found that over half of those surveyed said they look to the Internet first for health information before seeing their doctor.[11]

This trend creates additional work demands for PCPs, since the Pew study found that only 18 percent of individuals seeking health information on the

Web used the online information instead of going to see a physician.[12] The remainder, we may assume, both sought Web information and proceeded to see a physician at some point. More patients walking into the exam room having already gone online for information about various diseases and treatments (the two most common reasons found by Pew for patients going on the Web) means more time needed during the encounter to put any consumer-obtained information into its proper context, more time needed to debunk erroneous information, and more time to convince the patient that the physician's opinion counts more than anything they might find online.

Given a fifteen-minute average patient office visit, these situations are an added distraction for PCPs in their interactions with patients and can lower both the quality and length of communication time between the two groups during the visit. Most importantly, "empowered" patients may signal a wavering sense of trust in PCPs, a trust these professionals must then work harder to build in a work context they cannot control very well.

> This is the "microwave" generation. Everyone wants a quick fix now. Everyone wants to pop something into the microwave and you're done in fifteen or twenty seconds. They don't want to wait things out. Everybody wants everything done instantly. It makes our job tougher. I like patients who want to challenge me, who want to be part of their care. But there's a loss of respect for the doctor, the amount of knowledge we have, all the training we've put up with. That's more of a frustration, a challenge. No one really ever challenged you years ago. (Gary, internist)

While all PCPs thought this change tended to complicate or extend the actual patient visit, most also believed that there was a longer-term, positive effect that lasted well beyond that visit. Tony, an internist in his mid-fifties, talked about how, in the end, he liked that the Internet led to better-informed patients who could take more personal responsibility for their own care:

> I get a lot of patients who come in here with their Internet printouts, diagnosing what they already think they have. I have to also take the time to work with patients for whom I prescribe a drug and then they go home and go onto the Internet and say, "I'm not taking that." But I'd rather have a patient who's involved in their own care and interested rather than just blind allegiance, like it was when I first started out. I want somebody who has a vested interest in getting it right, because it gives me a chance to put some of the burden of improvement on them. If they're merely a submissive participant, then the entire burden of

everything is on me. Whereas if they're empowered by the virtue of the information available to them, to help in their own care, then I can expect them to participate in their own care, and follow my directions. If you've vetted the drug I've given you on the Internet, and I have your tacit approval, then I expect you to take the drug. If you've gone through the process, and I've passed your filter, then take my drug. But it's a double-edged sword. Some of the most commonly used medications in the world have Internet-labeled side-effects that are three pages long. One of the problems with Internet information is it's not put into con-text. You get the same bold-faced headlines for something that's one of a million complications as one of a thousand. That's where the physician's expertise is supposed to come in. But there is time and resources that have to be expended to do that, and you don't get paid to do that kind of education with patients. I feel that if you're going to prescribe a test or drug or procedure, you have to convince them it's valid and answer their questions. All these types of things weren't issues back then. It was simpler. (Tony, internist)

Paperwork Demands and the Double-Edged Sword of Technology

Another major change in the PCP workday is the amount of noncompensated time spent on administrative paperwork. Although more physicians found themselves under the protective umbrella of corporate practices, they still could not evade demands that required their personal review, professional opinion, approval, or signature.

For every hour I spend with patients, there's probably another fifteen to twenty minutes of administrative work created for myself. So, if you see patients eight hours a day, you're going to have another two hours of stuff to do on top of that. You don't get paid for that other stuff. And no one else can do it but you. (Charlie, family physician)

The PCPs' paperwork included gaining insurance approvals for patients to receive services and tests, dealing with insurers looking to trade one prescrip-tion drug for another cheaper one, handling over-the-phone patient requests for services like prescription refills, and reading the summaries sent by specialists whom patients had visited. While practice nursing staff may help in the logis-tical aspects of this administrative work, and may handle directly simpler issues, PCPs still must review everything that accompanies their ultimate sig-nature on a document. In many instances, such as with service denials from insurers or revised prescriptions in pharmacies, it is the physician who is required legally to deal directly with the matter. And the modification of clinical care decisions is the sole responsibility of the physician in a primary care practice.

> There are a lot of things that intrude on my day today that didn't back then. For example, today I must've gotten twenty-five faxes from pharmacy benefit companies requesting that I substitute this brand of drug, which my patients have been on for years, with this other one. Each one of those faxes requires my attention, and if I agree with it, then there is a patient call that's generated afterwards. I then get interrupted two or three times taking a call from a radiologist in California who has questions about my precertification for an imaging study I've ordered for a patient. And this is all outside of the confines of my interaction with the patient, and all unreimbursed time. I have to answer my office manager's question about why such and such a claim was denied, I have to write this letter of appeal to the insurance companies. (Tony, internist)

. . .

> We get a big, big volume of information from other specialists, and even more intrusion on our practice by the insurance companies. You get a letter from the insurance company that says, "Mr. Jones has diabetes and we can't find out whether he had an A1C in the last six months." So what do you do with that? We take the time to go to the chart—though that's not reimbursed—takes a lot of time. And a lot of times you find out, yes he had that test several times, it's just that it didn't get into the chart, it didn't get into the databank of the insurance company for some reason. We end up now with a big volume of paper flow even though we have an electronic medical record. A lot of time is spent handling this kind of stuff. Much more effort than twenty-five years ago. (Rose, internist)

. . .

> I spend a lot more time now fighting. Fighting with insurance companies. Fighting with drug formularies. I spend a lot more time doing administrative stuff because, for example, the patient is on a drug and their employer's just changed their insurance from this plan to another plan and now I have to change their medications because the plans each have their own drugs they reimburse. Or, some insurance plan now decides they're going to do precertification and I have to talk to some idiot behind a desk who won't let me do a CT-scan on a patient because

he thinks he knows what's going on. I spend lots of times checking formularies to see if the drug I want to put the patient on is on the list so it can get paid for. I spend a lot of time talking with pharmacies telling me that this drug is now off the formulary list and I have to find another one for the patient. (Rick, internist)

. . .

There are tons of regulations now, tons of insurance paperwork you have to deal with. Nothing's simple. Before, you could spend pretty much all of the fifteen minutes talking with the patient. Now you have to spend part of that time making sure all the documentation is there, you have to make sure the billing is in order, you have to keep track of any of the specialist care that's going on and review that first, make sure nothing is missed. All that before you start talking with the patient. (Loretta, family physician)

. . .

I have a stack of papers at the end of the day I have to fill out. I have names of parents I need to call. And I can't do that during the workday. Because I don't get paid for it. It doesn't generate income for the practice. So I do it at night and on the weekends. And some of the people I call will say, "It's Saturday, aren't you closed today?" (Peter, pediatrician)

PCPs talked about their paperwork and care coordination burdens as "nonrevenue generating" activities. This devalued them significantly. They understood it was expected by others as part of their job, and that proper execution of these activities was vital for helping patients get what they needed in a fragmented health care system. But most PCPs hated not getting paid to do it. There was resentment that came through in the way most talked that made it seem as if these activities could potentially be performed by PCPs in less than desirable ways for the patient. For some, it created negative attitudes toward patients.

You know, every minute of a lawyer's time is billable. Someone has to pay for it. If they talk to you on the phone for five minutes, well that's five minutes of their time and they're going to send you a bill for that. And you're going to pay it if you want to continue to do business with them. But people just expect doctors to give their time away for free. It's funny how no one sees the differences here. (Tony, internist)

. . .

Every time you interact with an attorney, if there's a phone call or an e-mail, you get charged. In my day, there's probably four hours easy that isn't billable. And the patient doesn't understand that. But most of it, things like workers comp forms, insurance approvals, whatever, it's done for them. (Quentin, family physician)

What made it worse for some PCPs was their feeling that these nonpaying demands created patient expectations that physicians could regularly do things for which they did not receive compensation:

> Patients want a lot of things to be done over the phone. Oftentimes, they want to avoid coming into the office if they can because they don't want to pay a co-pay. My time is valuable, and I don't get reimbursed for speaking on the phone with you, and if you want to have an in-depth discussion of a problem with me, or you want me to fill out paperwork for you, or you want a refill on your three-month Xanax prescription, then you're going to have to schedule an office visit, have a face-to-face meeting with me, pay your co-pay, and I will give you my undivided time during that office visit. They don't get the connection that if they don't come into the office, I don't get paid. (Sal, internist)

The care coordination demands imposed upon the PCP in the early twenty-first century deserve special mention here. The meaning of "care coordination" in primary care has evolved over time into something difficult to fulfill in practice. In theory, it is the opportunity for a patient to have a single clinician serving as the central repository for clinical information and decision making. This would be a clinician who advises patients on their myriad care needs and helps them navigate a fragmented health care system. This theoretical definition was very important to all PCPs in the study. No one doubted that such a role was valuable for the patient, and was ideally suited to them as primary care doctors.

However, in practice most PCPs felt that they were coordinators more in an administrative than clinical sense. They felt themselves to be the "dumping ground" used by specialists after the latter had seen the patient for their ultra-specific complaint or problem, addressed it, and then did not feel any further commitment to the patient. Most PCPs talked of their care-coordination roles as "physicians of last resort" who helped patients decipher the dense jargon of specialty medicine, deal with impersonal specialists, and compile a variety of different physician notes and hospital discharge summaries into a coherent whole that provided a clear timeline and summation of the patient's clinical situation.

> Down the line, if I have very sick patients who are seeing specialists for management of critical issues, am I still managing those things? No. But those patients are still going to come back to me and say, "I don't know

what that guy just said. I didn't like him at all. Could you please put this in plain English for me." (Wilma, family physician)

. . .

I must get two-hundred pieces of paper every few days, and some are patient discharge summaries from hospital stays and specialist notes, some of which I didn't even know about because I didn't even know the patient had gone to see a specialist. But once the specialist is finished caring for that patient's specific problem, they send them right back to me. If the patient says to the specialist, "Well, Doc, what about my diabetes, could it be related to this problem?" the specialist says, "I don't know, you need to go to your primary care doctor and ask him about that." They have no interest in seeing the whole patient. So they deal with what they need to deal with, and then send me their conclusions. Then the patient looks to me to make sense of it all. When a lot of times they didn't even ask me if they should see that specialist in the first place. (Mark, internist)

PCPs spoke of care coordination as a largely noncompensated set of activities. While they recognized how valuable their role was in being the "go-to" physician for patients, especially when something serious presented in their office, they spoke with ambivalence about the lack of external recognition of that role by insurers and colleagues.

Twenty-five years ago, a patient came in with chest pain, you did a chest X-ray, there's a spot on their lung, you admit them to the hospital, a surgeon would see them and do a biopsy. I had a patient come in here today who had a chest X-ray two days ago, a CT scan one day ago, showed an abnormality, I sent that patient to a surgeon today, and they biopsied that patient today. So, within forty-eight hours without hitting the hospital, we have a diagnosis. But it took a lot of arranging to get to that point, to the diagnosis. Twenty-five years ago that would have been a hospitalization for a week. It would have been a protracted process. Here it was a lot of resources spent by the primary care office in arranging for the tests, getting the test results, discussing the test results with the patient, calling the consultant, and getting the patient over there. There are a lot of steps in that. OK? And we billed probably a $60 or $70 office visit for that. That kind of involvement for a primary care physician to make a diagnosis, get that patient to the right place, it takes some skills, takes some training, takes access to the testing that wasn't even available years ago. (Barry, internist)

One of the most profound changes that stand to transform the physician's office and patient care is the electronic medical record (EMR). EMRs have been lauded by insurers, government, employers, and clinicians as vital for improving quality of care and patient satisfaction. Advantages identified include greater integration between specialist and primary care, enhanced communication, more efficient care delivery, and patient empowerment. Despite these highly touted benefits, a smaller number of primary care physicians use any type of EMR. Moreover, EMRs have been shown not to be foolproof improvers of efficiency or quality.[13] Still, a majority of PCPs in the current study had either already made the transition to an EMR system or were planning to do so in the near future, in large part because the organizations in which they were employed believed that there would be cost savings and higher-quality care from using these systems.

PCPs as a whole were less enthusiastic about the critical role of an EMR system in their everyday work lives. Above all else, most believed it did not automatically make their work simpler or more efficient, nor did it necessarily improve quality of care in significant ways from their points of view. Wanda is a midcareer pediatrician who works in a practice with three other physicians. Her practice is part of a larger primary care business entity that has over seventy physicians working for it. The company has slowly phased in the introduction of electronic medical records over a two-year period. Technically savvy and willing to incorporate new methods into her practice, Wanda was a big proponent of the move from paper to electronic charts. But that enthusiasm waned with her experiences watching how providers interact with the EMR.

I don't really care for the EMR system we have. It doesn't save us time. And there are in theory a lot of advantages to it. I was in favor of using it, because I felt there were a lot of opportunities to improve care, like cross-checking on patients and flagging ones that needed certain things done at a given time. And there's a lot of potential for better documentation. But in the particular system we have, it's just so tedious. You have to click-click-click-click probably fifty times just to write a clinical note. It's ridiculous. And part of it is how it was designed and implemented. There are templates and none of them really fit pediatrics.

So you constantly have to change the template if you want to use it. To take out the stuff that's not appropriate for that particular age. It's an EMR intended for the whole company, which includes a lot of different specialties. And the IT people are like, "Yeah, but it can do this and do that!" And I say, "Yeah, but if you do that every time you'll be here until

10 P.M. every day." As it is, we've been doing it for almost two years, and it's still very tedious for most of us. And some of the older docs just use the bare minimum of it to get by, just to get it done, so that when you read the clinical notes they write, you're like, "What the hell is this?" There's no information. Because they don't fill stuff in.

And if you use it like it should be used, it should make things more accurate and specifically defined and more documented. However, there's also the temptation, and I've seen it many, many times in our own practice, to just click on a standard visit link, like "Brief-Normal Visit," which then pulls up this whole exam which includes all these different things you check and fill in, for nothing more than an ear infection, let's say, if that's what the patient has. You don't check things like the thyroid for an ear infection, but it's still there on the standard template. But because it's tedious to erase all those standard items, you don't, and then the electronic documentation shows that you did this stuff, because you didn't take the time to erase it for that visit on the template. And so, you click on "ear infection" and put that in as the diagnosis, but then all of the template goes into the patient record as if you did it all. To me, that's a big problem. It's just tempting with these things to click and go, when it's not an accurate representation of the exam you did.

When you have a certain number of patients you have to see, and a certain number of notes to get done, what are you going to do, take the time to change around every template? That takes a lot of time, and you either run behind or, if you wait until the end of the day to do it, it keeps you here or you're doing it at home. Like for me, I'd go home and take care of my daughter, put her to bed, and then I'm logging into the EMR system at 11 at night to do my notes for the day. (Wanda, pediatrician)

Wanda's indictment of her practice's EMR system was supported by other PCPs, a few of whom worked with the same system as Wanda, and the rest in practices that had different EMR systems. All of these were physicians who had been working with an EMR system for several years, so their perceptions were not shaped by the newness of their experience with the technology. Similar to all the discussions was the recognition by PCPs that an EMR shaped the ways in which clinicians communicated the pertinent facts of a given patient visit. For some, it took much more time to enter information into an EMR than on a paper chart.

The most challenging thing to the EMR is getting the [patient] notes in. It helps a lot with things like keeping track of prescriptions, ordering prescriptions, and sending them direct to the pharmacy. But it takes longer to get notes into the system. There are different types of visits. Some are easier to do on computer, say like a sore throat where you have a few check marks to make and it's "boom, boom, boom." Other things like an adult with multiple problems, the templates we have on the computer don't work well for that. So a lot of that has to become free text where you're typing everything in. And I'm not the best typist so it takes me a while to get things done. (Greg, internist and pediatrician)

Many PCPs felt that the EMR created a threat of greater inaccuracy in documenting the specific events of a patient encounter. A big part of this was not having enough time to edit standard templates or write full visit notes. Quentin, a midcareer family practitioner, had also lost faith in the value of the EMR as a communications tool.

Part of what makes my workday longer is the electronic medical record, which I think for a lot of people has become a pain. It's very time consuming. And the benefits from the point of view of increased quality, I don't see. There are some very small benefits with respect to prescriptions, but in almost every other respect the chart is less meaningful. It's a bunch of templates, and what you end up seeing in those templates may not even be accurate. If all you do with these templates on the EMR is just push a button, the information may not be accurate. I may or may not do things exactly the way it's laid out in the template, for a physical exam, say. And I try and go back and change the template or make the corrections of what I did do. But I may not do it 100 percent. Or, if I'm rushed or pressed for time and I go back six hours later, I may not remember what I did with complete certainty. Whereas if I'm dictating something, and I'm doing it during or immediately after the visit, it's what I did and what I saw or observed. There's a tendency with the computerized record to have things pop out at you and this also stifles your own thinking, makes you respond to what the EMR is asking you for rather than you telling the EMR what you feel is relevant to put into the record, what's the key insight you got from talking with the patient or examining them. (Quentin, family physician)

Mark, an internist, felt that use of an EMR contributed to a pattern of doctors in all specialties who are less willing to commit the time or focus to writing a detailed visit note. For him, getting patient information quicker from an EMR compared to a written chart had to be weighed against the potential "voltage drop" in the usefulness of the information contained in the electronic record.

> The electronic medical record is both a boon and a bane. It is a boon because it makes information much more readily accessible, which is the important part. As such, I think it does improve quality of care for some things, but not all of them. The bane is that, harkening back to an age when people spoke to one another in person, or when people wrote instead of text messaged in abbreviated code, doctors used to set down their mindset in their clinical note. And you could read a consultation, perhaps glean information that you hadn't gotten before about the patient, gain a new insight. It was a narrative, a story. It was pleasant to read the story, someone else's assessment as to why they thought it was rheumatoid arthritis as opposed to mixed connective tissue disease. When people fill out a note electronically, you get much less of that story. And so you get much less potential for the new insight or knowing why the other doctor concluded things the way he did. (Mark, internist)

The views expressed by Wanda, Quentin, Mark, Gary, and other PCPs in the study raise interesting insights about the value of an electronic medical record for patient care. In an industrial society such as ours, the assumption is that more or advanced technology is always better, and that assumption certainly is one made unfailingly in the health care industry. At times, it is accurate. There is little doubt that the use of electronic medical records which force different physicians to input similar data in standardized ways enhances care on a population-based level—for example, all patients in a primary care network. It allows for the kinds of widespread performance monitoring and patient risk identification that improves health care quality. It produces data and reports that create greater transparency and accountability in how care is delivered, by comparing physicians against one another and against approved care standards. It also may reduce errors in areas like drug prescribing, where computerized order entry reduces the potential for illegible handwriting to be misread and the wrong prescriptions filled.

Yet, most of the PCPs in the study who had been using EMRs for several years did not buy into the EMR concept because of parochial concerns that focused on how the technology complicated their workday. They evaluated the change from paper to electronic patient records in terms of whether or not it created more work for them, and whether or not they felt satisfied, in terms of their own standards, about the type of patient and visit information contained in the EMR. It was clear that not all PCPs trusted one another, or other types of physicians, to guard against the pitfalls that might produce an inaccurate or incomplete electronic patient record. This lack of trust derived from their experiences using the EMR, which involved watching what their colleagues did, and perhaps their own behaviors that were consistent with the very problems they illuminated. In either case, the experiences themselves were linked to a hectic, fast-paced workday that was not ameliorated by the presence of the EMR system, a workday whose focus on generating billable visits made using an EMR for higher-quality care a difficult luxury to pursue.

Chapter 4

Leaving Hospital Work Behind

Fewer primary care physicians do any type of hospital-based medicine today. If current trends hold, there may be no primary care physicians who provide both hospital and office-based care. Hospital medicine involves taking care of patients in the hospital when they are sick enough to warrant inpatient care and monitoring. Hospitalization may occur for a range of conditions and needed services including heart failure, general and specialty surgery, cardiac bypass surgery, infections, pneumonia, diabetes complications, falls and fractures, joint replacements, and cancer care. It also involves geriatric care for elderly patients experiencing acute episodes that require a hospital stay.

Caring for their patients when they were in the hospital used to be a normal part of every PCP's workday.

> Twenty-five years ago, when I started this, as a primary care physician I would go to the hospital at 7 or 8 every morning, make rounds until 10 or 11 A.M., come into the office and see patients until dinnertime, and that was my day. If something happened with a hospital patient that required me to stop back into the hospital in the evening, then I did that too. (Barry, internist)

Up to five years ago, hospital medicine had a central place of importance in the daily work life of a PCP. This importance derived out of the view of PCPs as true generalists, caring for their patients in sickness and health. This view was appropriate before the advent of physician specialists trained to care only for select diseases. It also fit better in a time when the amount of clinical knowledge needed to manage hospitalizations was much less than it is today.

Hospitals now contain only the very sick. Beginning with the advent of a funding formula called "Diagnostic Related Groupings" (DRG) over two decades ago, hospitals have decreased the number of inpatient beds they maintain while shortening the length of stay for all hospitalizations.

> More patients are being kept out of the hospital than ever before. In 1978, I was the Associate Director of Medicine at [the local] hospital. In 1978, there were 150,000 hospital days there. I think last year there were probably 50,000 days. (Barry, internist)

The DRGs set reimbursement for hospital care on a prospective basis, the dollars fixed based on the patient's clinical diagnosis. This prevented hospitals from charging whatever they wished for a hospital stay, as they had been used to doing. When hospitals could set their own rates, often the same services were priced much differently across hospitals, for no good reason, and there was no incentive to be cost-efficient in how care was provided. There was also an incentive to keep patients in the hospital for as long as possible, resulting in lower quality of care. The DRGs changed all of this by providing hospitals with an incentive to provide services in a manner that fixed the patients' problems yet discharged them quickly.

The evolution of medical science and technology has also played a major part in decreasing demand for inpatient hospital services. The development of quick, definitive diagnostic technologies such as CT scans and magnetic resonance imaging (MRI) make many diagnoses possible in the outpatient setting. This avoids a hospital stay for the patient. In addition, enhanced knowledge of disease processes related to diabetes, hypertension, heart failure, and all forms of cancer have produced more effective treatments that lessen a patient's morbidity and mortality. Modern medicine now prevents many disease complications that traditionally would have required lengthy stays in the hospital.

Even most surgeries can now be done outside of the hospital through ambulatory surgery centers often attached directly to specialist offices. Surgeries that required four and five days of stay, or longer, are now often completed the same or next day, allowing the patient to go home quickly. In short, our need for the hospital is much less than thirty or forty years ago. This fact is reflected in the statistical paradox that while more people in the United States have chronic disease diagnoses than ever before, and are living longer, hospital length of stay has decreased significantly for almost every age group in society. Between 1970 and 2005, average hospital length of stay decreased 2 days for ages fifteen to forty-four, 4.3 days for forty-five to sixty-four-year-olds, and more than 7 days for these age sixty-five and over.[1] Across all age groups, hospital stays were 3 days less in 2005 compared to 1970.

The fledgling specialty of hospital medicine has helped drain the pool of eligible primary care doctors, since hospitalists draw heavily on the ranks of internal medicine and pediatric residents. The fit of hospital medicine with internal medicine and pediatric residency training is ideal. Most of these residencies are based primarily in hospital settings, and residents in both areas spend a great deal of their work time caring for inpatients. Because of heavy inpatient work experience, these young doctors are better groomed initially to work as hospitalists than as office-based primary care physicians. So it is no surprise that for many young primary care residents, hospital medicine is a natural career choice.

> My residency training prepared me better to take care of sick kids than healthy kids. That was one of my challenges when I started working after residency. I was overwhelmed by my lack of preparedness for being a primary care physician, seeing patients in an office setting. When I started out, I could take care of a thirty-two-week premature infant with respiratory distress with one arm tied behind my back, that's how much neonatal intensive care unit exposure I had in my training. But if you gave me a three-year-old having temper tantrums, I wouldn't have had the faintest idea of what to tell the parents, because I wasn't exposed to much of that in my training. (Peter, pediatrician)

> . . .

> We have so many requirements we have to fill in our residency programs, that by the end of three years we do not get enough primary care exposure, enough exposure to ambulatory care settings and office practice. We do once a year a month-block of primary care. The rest of the time it's twice a week. And a lot of it is almost like urgent care, in the sense that it's patients I may have not seen before, they have acute things, they need the clinic to get taken care of, so I have to get them in, treat them, and get them out. There's not really a lot of continuity of care I can do, or do physicals or preventive stuff. And my friends' internal medicine programs have even less outpatient primary care. We are all so trained and comfortable with inpatient medicine that come July 1, when we graduate from residency, after our three years, all we know is inpatient medicine. That's what we are comfortable with. So more general internists are looking to become hospitalists because it's very similar to what they've done for the past three years. Even when I'm in the primary care clinic we do here, when I see something like a rash I have to call the

attending in because, honestly, how many rashes have I seen? While here in the hospital if I see cellulitis, it wouldn't take me more than two seconds to say, "Hey, that's cellulitis, let's start antibiotics." (Pam, internist)

Of the entire sample of out-of-residency PCPs interviewed, less than ten were still doing any type of hospital care. PCPs still doing hospital care did it at a reduced rate—either as part of an academic or teaching position they maintained, or to remain symbolically connected to the hospital for the sake of their patients. The rest had given over their hospital duties to a hospitalist or hospitalist group. For the PCPs working in larger primary care networks, this was a business decision, hoisted on them by the network itself. For others, it was also a business decision, but one freely chosen to enhance their fiscal viability by generating additional office visit revenue.

It just doesn't make a lot of economic sense for me to go to this hospital and see my one patient in the morning, then drive over to this other hospital and see my two patients there, then get into the office later and have to stay later just to make up for the patient visits I missed in the office. (Rick, internist)

. . .

Five years ago, our practice was probably 60 percent outpatient, and 40 percent inpatient. And as of two years ago, we got out of the hospital altogether. Not because we didn't like the hospital. But because economically the hospital took so much time, and the reimbursement so poor, that you could be in your office and make enough to survive whereas you couldn't in the hospital setting. So, we came up with a system to solve that, and the way we solved that was to contract with a hospitalist group who takes care of our patients as inpatients, and then we stay in the office all day and see our patients when they come back [from the hospital]. (Francis, family physician)

. . .

I don't work in the hospital anymore, which is a change from how it used to be. But it's a necessity. I can make more money coming into the office and seeing patients all morning than I can going to the hospital to see my one or two patients there. It's a change, and there are trade-offs. (Gary, internist)

Every PCP in the study appreciated the business-related benefits of having someone available to the practice that cares for sick inpatients all day long. There was a clear level of acceptance of the hospitalist need among all the

PCPs, which is consistent with the published research.[2] It made their daily work lives easier and more predictable. It allowed them to focus on their office practice and take advantage of the incentives in that environment.

> I was doing hospital rounding up until about a year ago. The other partners in my group decided to give this up to a hospital group several years ago, and I was the only one left rounding. Being the only one left doing this in the practice, it became increasingly difficult to maintain this schedule, especially with the need to have a full patient load in the office. My schedule is a bit easier now. I don't have to worry about getting up early and going to the hospital to round on people or deal with an admission. I don't have to rush to the office anymore or run back to the hospital to deal with something during the day. (Sal, internist)
>
> . . .
>
> I spent so much more time in the hospital than I got paid for. I mean, I would spend hours sometimes in a given day, because I wanted my patients to get what they needed, but it just didn't make sense from the standpoint of earning a living. (Loretta, family physician)

Giving up hospital medicine made a lot of sense when considering the economic imperative under which PCPs now operated. It was the fiscally smart thing to do in a field where reimbursements had become tied to office visits, patient panels were larger and more demanding, and practice overhead was costlier because of new demands around quality of care and the use of technology. PCPs in the study started seeing patients in the office at eight or nine in the morning because they no longer had to spend two hours at the hospital. They could see twenty-five to thirty patients in the office in a given day, tend to their paperwork demands, and still make it home by six or seven each night. They could set up their ambulatory care workday knowing that they would have no interruptions generated by patients showing up in the hospital emergency room, patients already in the hospital developing complications, or patients being discharged from the hospital. Getting rid of hospital care purified their workday in the sense that it allowed them to focus singularly on the individuals that moved through their office exam rooms.

Deskilling and the PCP Who Does Not Do Hospital Care

Despite these clear economic benefits, though, how some PCPs talked about the sacrifice of hospital work conjured up images of professional deskilling for the field of primary care. This deskilling resulted from individual PCPs no longer performing a complex component of medical work—hospital medicine—

handing that work over to another physician group, and replacing it with office work that in many instances required less skill and task variety. Deskilling often results from seemingly rational decisions to improve the efficiency and quality associated with a given production process. The labor in that production process becomes highly specialized, focused only on doing one part of it competently, but then over time grows less able to perform a variety of jobs in the process, losing occupational prestige and autonomy as a result.

Even when considering the economic benefits, why would this group so quickly and easily give up the most important part of what made it unique as a field of medicine, that is, the ability to provide full continuity of care for individuals through all stages of health and illness? After all, no other physician group in American medicine can make this same continuity claim. And would the decision to give up hospital medicine be one they would collectively come to regret, especially if it weakened their knowledge base, legitimacy with patients, and prestige as a professional group?

Brian is a family physician in his early fifties who still does hospital medicine and delivers babies, as well as manages a full schedule of office-based care each day. While he thought the reasons for why doctors might give up hospital care were fairly simple, and extended beyond just the business case and into the lifestyle realm, he also felt that the collective impact of such a decision on PCPs was serious.

> I understand why you wouldn't want to do hospital medicine. Who wants to get up at 2 A.M. in the morning to go to the hospital? If you don't do hospital work, you have a lot more control over your schedule. When you say to your spouse you'll be home for dinner, you almost assuredly will be home for dinner. There's less hassle, more uninterrupted sleep. Who can argue that? But I still do the hospital, I still deliver babies. I think you lose a part of yourself when you don't do hospital medicine. You go to the hospital and see one of your patients, and you see them brighten up right before your eyes. You can't put a price on that.
>
> I worry about what will happen if we give that up. We've always been so linked to the hospital. What I worry about is that there will be this "town-gown" mentality—you'll have the people who work in the hospital that are considered "high-tech." And the doctors working in the community who are the "lower-tech" and just like it has developed in other countries, the community doctors won't have the same access to information and expertise, nor will they get the same respect as those working in the hospital. (Brian, family physician)

Comments like Brian's pushed me to listen intently to how PCPs thought about and experienced the sacrifice of hospital work in their everyday work lives. What were they really giving up? Were they at all concerned that it could undermine their authority with patients and standing relative to the rest of the medical profession? Was this idea of an "easier" work life thanks to the absence of hospital medicine widespread? On the surface, PCPs touched upon the topic of giving up hospital medicine tangentially, either in describing their typical workday or as a point of clarification that might be useful to me. But it soon became clear as I probed further that many PCPs struggled with how to interpret the absence of hospital work in the context of their roles as doctors.

For example, Paul was a young, bright family physician who still did a week of hospital care every six weeks as part of a teaching position in his former residency program. However, he did no hospital care in his other part-time, office-based job for a large primary care practice network. Paul struggled with how to think about the pros and cons of this collective decision that the field of primary care now embraced. He could not personally imagine at this early point in his career not doing at least some hospital medicine. He trained in a hospital setting during residency. It seemed both natural and expected to take care of his patients when they were sickest. But he had conflicting feelings related to how much hospital work he could do and still feel competent at it, and he acknowledged that more hospital work might undermine his desire for a balanced lifestyle.

> You have to realize hospital work is a lot. You're going in, checking labs, talking with nurses and specialists, coordinating the care in terms of what's going on, writing your note. It's not a quick thing. The problem is, when you step away from it for awhile, you can tend to shy away from it. You say to yourself, "Ooh, I haven't taken care of a patient in the hospital for awhile. And for me, even, not doing OB anymore since residency, I don't do the deliveries anymore, you start to feel gun shy. I think it's harder if you're not doing a lot of it, to go back to it. I do the hospital only every six weeks, and I still say to myself every six weeks, "Well, here I go, it's been six weeks." I always feel a bit hesitant, like I'm not going to do a good job. I can imagine if you don't do it at all, you're going to be intimidated by having not done it for awhile. My wife is a physician, too. And we have a newborn baby that we both want to spend time with. Having the time for my family is very important to me, and so not doing hospital work helps me have more time with my family, which is a good thing. (Paul, internist)

Sarah was a general internist in her early thirties who had recently relocated to the area. She had worked full-time doing hospital-based primary care before beginning her new job as a suburban doctor in a group practice that still did a small portion of its own hospital care. Sarah was interested in maintaining some sort of presence in the hospital. She also felt there were meaningful benefits for her own professional development.

> You learn things in the hospital where even if you never practice hospital medicine, it's good to know them. It's good to be able to describe to the patient, for example, what the machine looks like and how it works when they're going to get a stress test. In the hospital, you learn a lot about the subspecialties, which as a primary care doc you need to know to be proficient. Either to know who to refer to and when, or know what to do yourself. Also, from the patient's perspective, there's nothing better than seeing their doctor in the hospital every day. The patient knows you. You know the patient. (Sarah, internist)

Sarah also had an infant at home and worked part-time. When pressed, she did not express much remorse about her current reality of doing almost no hospital work. Both Paul and Sarah appreciated the reality that their patients would prefer seeing them in the hospital, as did all the PCPs in the study. However, neither Paul nor Sarah nor any of the younger PCPs in the study regretted a reduced or nonexistent role in hospital medicine. This was surprising at first glance, since these doctors were not far removed from residency experiences that placed hospital care at the center of their everyday lives. However, when considered in the context of their own strong feelings that hospital work complicated a PCP's everyday work life, made it difficult to generate an adequate income, and created more night and weekend work duties that detracted from a good lifestyle, it became an easier decision to make.

> I personally was not a big fan of the hospital. I enjoyed doing it during residency, but I didn't see myself working in an office and getting twenty phone calls a day from the hospital for this, that, or the other thing. I truly enjoy the fact that we have a hospitalist who works for us because it makes my day flow more smoothly. You don't have to stop when someone's having chest pain and drive to the hospital and come back an hour later. That's the positive aspect. The negative aspect is that for the patients you develop a relationship with, you don't get to see them when they are in the hospital because they are being covered by somebody else. I'm friends with a family, and I had their grandfather as my patient,

and he just passed away. And the friends would call me every couple of days and give me updates on the grandfather. And they would say, "Boy, I really wish you could spend more time in the hospital." So, I understand why patients would say that, but they also don't understand how much it upsets the work flow and your own schedule if you were to do that. Not doing the hospital keeps me flowing smoothly and allows me to have a family life. (Harry, internist)

Similar to many young doctors in the study, Paul and Sarah wanted a balanced lifestyle as much as anything else in their careers. Lifestyle is the twenty-first-century mantra of many new physicians. The biggest upside of not doing hospital medicine was the chance to attain this balance without sacrificing income or devoting more time to work. Hospital care required getting up an hour or two earlier each day, getting into the office later in the morning, leaving for home later in the day, more call responsibilities, and late-night calls from patients and hospital emergency departments for new admissions. In many ways, it was the enemy of a balanced lifestyle.

The Intangibles of Doing Hospital Work

Older PCPs doing hospital work for most of their careers were more wistful about what its absence meant for them. Like younger PCPs, they also accepted it as an economic imperative. But unlike younger physicians, doing hospital work had been an accepted job requirement that shaped their identities as professionals. They viewed the lifestyle implications of hospital work less negatively than younger PCPs, since they had long ago adapted their lives to the realities of workdays with the hospital as part of their obligation. Issues viewed negatively by younger PCPs, such as starting work earlier or going home later, were not emphasized by older PCPs, although they acknowledged that there were nice lifestyle by-products that went with not having to go to the hospital on a regular basis.

Instead, older PCPs emphasized hospital work issues that came from the experiences of having done them on a regular basis for years. Because of their lack of involvement in hospital medicine, younger doctors emphasized more of what they gained by not doing hospital medicine, while older doctors, because of years of hospital work experience, emphasized what they lost when giving it up. Tony is a general internist in his late fifties who was one of the few PCPs interviewed still treating patients in the hospital. His other practice partners had already given their hospital work over to a hospitalist group. Tony was the last holdout.

I find it very intellectually satisfying to take care of sick patients. To interact with different people—specialists, nurses, technicians—all taking care of a sicker patient in the hospital. If you can take someone who walks into the hospital very ill, and you help them walk out better, that's very rewarding. And the hospitalist model does away with that. Much of primary care is routine, everyday common illness. It's important, but it's routine and common. And my feeling is that as an internist if the diseases I see day in and day out—diabetes, hypertension, obesity, muscular pain—the routine, everyday things that pop up, if I have to do that every single day, go to work every day knowing the faces may change, the names may change, but I'll be doing the exact same thing everyday, then how does that make me any different from someone on an assembly line, screwing in the same bolt? The car may be different, but the bolt is the same. If I had to do the same thing every day, I'd be bored to death. Now that appeals to some people, who want to start and end their day at predictable times. But it doesn't appeal to me. (Tony, internist)

Mark, also an internist in his fifties, continued to do hospital medicine but at a reduced rate. Neither he nor his partners were willing to turn over complete care of their hospital-bound patients to hospitalists. Mark spoke of the traditional place of hospital medicine in the PCP's workday. Like most mid- and later-career PCPs, he believed that doing hospital medicine was part of being a well-rounded doctor. He also raised another drawback of no longer doing hospital medicine: the decreased social interaction it produced with specialists such as cardiologists, surgeons, emergency medicine physicians, and critical care physicians—all of whom worked mostly in hospital settings. This social interaction created camaraderie for PCPs with others not in their field and produced learning opportunities where they could gain knowledge and exposure to the latest clinical developments across a variety of medical areas.

That connection with other physicians, outside of the colleagues in your own office, is important. When I first went into practice, it wasn't unusual to hang around for awhile in the hospital after rounds were over, and talk to some of the docs. There was a grand rounds you could attend somewhere, at the medical college or hospital. People would share thoughts and presentations. You could dialogue with specialists on certain issues. We haven't done that stuff in a decade. Now, even though we are still doing our own hospital care, you have to get out of there and hit the ground running when you come into the office. There's no time anymore for those opportunities. You have to learn on your own.

> Leaving the hospital entirely scares us because it would be another tie
> that would be cut, that would lessen our ability to keep in touch with
> other doctors, with the advances in clinical medicine. (Mark, internist)

Tony echoed Mark's sentiments, but focused on how interaction with specialists through his work at the hospital enabled him to gain knowledge about
where to refer his patients, improving quality of care and achieving a better fit
between patient and specialist in the long run.

> If I didn't go to the hospital, there would be weeks that go by where I
> wouldn't interact with a specialist in a professional setting. I might go
> out to dinner with them, but I wouldn't interact with them in a clinical
> setting. When you're referring one of your patients to a specialist, you
> want to know what this person [the specialist] is like. I want to know
> more than just if they know how to tie knots or put tubes in someone.
> I want to know what kind of person they are because I try to match my
> referral physician to the temperament of the patient. If I know my
> patient needs a lot of hand-holding and bedside manner, I'll refer to a
> person who has good skills and those qualities as well, instead of some-
> one who just has good technical or diagnostic skills. And if I never inter-
> act with these people, how do I know? So, I don't think I'm doing my
> patient a service. (Tony, internist)

Theresa was a middle-aged family doctor who had recently joined a large
primary care practice network. She worked in a small rural primary care office
that belonged to the network. Theresa still did hospital work every day, regardless of whether she had one or five of her patients to visit at a given time. She did
not have plans to give it up because of fears of what she might lose in doing so.

> Giving up the hospital will make it more isolating for primary care docs.
> I mean, if I spent the whole day here and never went to the hospital,
> never interacted with specialists, didn't get involved in medical admin-
> istration stuff, committees and that kind of thing, I think I would become
> very isolated. I know some docs and they love it this way, but I think it's
> very isolating. When someone goes into the hospital, you punt them off
> until they come back to the office. I get tremendous satisfaction out of
> taking care of someone in the hospital, whom I've known for years, to
> assist with their care vis-à-vis specialists in the hospital, because the spe-
> cialists don't know the patient. The interaction with specialists is very
> important for my own professional growth and increasing my medical
> knowledge. But the personal satisfaction I get from that patient getting

better in the hospital and then going home to a productive life, just knowing that I've done the best I can as their personal physician. People feel like I care about them at every stage of their life. They don't have to feel like, "Oh, now I'm in the hospital and so she's going to write me off." Not the case at all. I stay actively involved when they're in the hospital. I get tremendous satisfaction from that. (Theresa, family physician)

Whether young or older, only a handful of PCPs linked their decisions not to do hospital medicine to larger implications for their field as a whole. Instead, PCP interviewees were concerned with how *not* doing hospital medicine might affect their daily work lives, skill sets, and patient relationships. However, in choosing to give up complex and clinically interesting work to others, and in transferring the care of their patients to other physicians at the moment those patients expected their support, PCPs left themselves open to a cruel irony: to remain economically viable and have a better lifestyle in the short run, they risked being seen as replaceable for other parts of their work besides hospital medicine—work that was less intense, complex, and important to the patient.

By acknowledging the advantages offered by hospitalists, they created openings for other groups such as nurse practitioners and physician assistants to offer themselves as viable alternatives for other parts of primary care work. Because if some of their most complex work could be reassigned to others easily, could not the same be done for their more routine work? PCPs did not seem to realize the active role they played in making this reality come true. Many still spoke of external forces, beyond their control, that made them give up hospital medicine without realizing their own culpability in making this choice, a choice that rendered their entire field less unique and prestigious. This deflecting of blame onto others was characteristic of how most PCPs talked about giving up hospital medicine.

The Effects on Patient Care and Relationships from Not Doing Hospital Work

Theresa's take on doing hospital medicine highlights two practically important questions raised by the trend of PCPs to no longer work in a hospital: what is the effect on patient care, and on the relationship between primary care physicians and their patients? Taken as a whole, the small amount of published research examining the quality of care and efficiency provided by hospitalists compared to PCPs in the management of hospital inpatients supports the conclusion that hospitalists likely provide as good, perhaps even more efficient clinical care than PCPs. Hospitalists have been shown to decrease patient length of stay. One literature review found that length of stay of hospitalists' patients decreased on average by 17 percent compared to these of PCPs.[3] This same review also found that hospitalists achieved average cost savings of approximately 13 percent per patient compared to PCPs.[4]

A 2005 review looking at over twenty separate published studies of hospitalists concluded that, overall, hospitalists reduce the cost of inpatient care, primarily due to a reduction in the length of stay rather than by providing fewer services, without negatively affecting quality of care or patient satisfaction.[5] A 2007 study published in the *New England Journal of Medicine* showed reduced lengths of stay for hospitals that use hospitalists compared to the use of both family practitioners and general internists, although the cost savings were marginal in one case and nonexistent in the other.[6]

A number of PCPs in the study thought hospitalists were an intelligent alternative. For example, Greg is an internist-pediatrician in his late forties who used to work in an academic medical center. For the past several years, he has worked for a large primary care network that employs hospitalists to take care of his patients.

> I think the hospitalist system is good, and I've been on both sides of it. The problem is being a primary care physician, when we'd admit a patient to the hospital, we'd see them for ten minutes in the morning, and be gone the rest of the day until the next morning. And what's here is what's here. So when you're in the office, your mind is not on the hospital or the patients there. You might order some tests in the morning but you wouldn't find out those results until the next day. It's hard to keep up with everything.
>
> Things have become much more complicated. More information and things to keep up on in your outpatient practice. Trying to keep up on hospital medicine as well is tough. We ended up figuring out that most of the patients we admitted needed a specialist anyway, so we ended up being basically secretaries, going to the hospital to see the patient but not really running the show like the specialists were. And the hospital we were admitting to was thirty or thirty-five minutes away, so if there was an emergency we could not be there in any amount of time to deal with it. I just don't think it's the best care for the patients. If you think about hospitalists, that's all they do—hospital medicine. Twenty-four hours a day. There's always someone in the hospital at least during business hours so if there's a change in condition or an emergency, they can respond to it. (Greg, internist and pediatrician)

Colin is a family physician who works for a rural practice.

> The hospitalists are quite solid. I have two sets that I work with, each at
> a different hospital. I can call them up and tell them that this or that
> patient is coming in. If there's something going on, they'll not infre-
> quently call me and say, "The patient's here, I wanted to give you a
> heads-up."

PCPs, especially the younger ones, appeared more willing to admit the
advantages of having someone available for inpatients at all times during the
day in the hospital, someone whose expertise was focused solely on treating
acutely ill individuals. Some younger PCPs conveyed an opinion that their own
involvement in hospital medicine added an unnecessary element of risk to
patient care. This risk came out of having them do something for which they
had less everyday experience and did sporadically. Hospital care is prone to
mistakes and errors given the level of illness experienced by patients and the
organizational complexity of hospital settings.[7]

> I'm fortunate, because in this practice we do not round on patients in the
> hospital. We just do outpatients. Which is absolutely fine by me. If our
> patients need to be admitted to a hospital, we recommend they go to hos-
> pitals with hospitalist services. For me, if I were doing it on my own,
> following my own patients in the hospital, right now I have no patients
> admitted, and you can have no patients admitted for several weeks. So,
> you are doing something that might be infrequent, which is not ideal for
> you or the patient, and there are these people who work in the hospital
> and that's all they do, take care of hospitalized patients, so they get bet-
> ter at it. (Lou, internist and pediatrician)

As I listened to these rational explanations from PCPs of why they thought
hospitalists could take care of their patients better than they could, I also read
into the explanations another strongly held belief—that doing hospital medicine on more than simply a token basis enhanced PCP skills and knowledge to
do their entire job, including office-based care.

> I think when you're taking care of patients in the hospital you gain
> insight into their disease process. You've got specialists and specialty
> care that you can see the nuances of that are different than what you're
> doing day to day. Mentally too it's different. When people are at their
> worst, other things come up that you may have not been privy to when
> you just see them in the office. You can get a whole different picture and

perspective on this person that you've known for a long time. I like that. It's important. (Paul, family physician)

. . .

You end up being a glorified physicians' assistant if you don't experience some level of hospital medicine in your work. Because it's not just about that fifteen minutes they're in your office and you're looking at them. There are other times too, and you're learning new things during those other times, things that enable you to understand the patient's state better. (Loretta, family physician)

. . .

You can't really know when to keep a patient out of the hospital until you know what it's like or how sick they are when they are in the hospital. And you get exposed to sickest patients in the hospital so when you don't have those experiences it detracts from your outpatient management to some degree. (Jane, family physician)

. . .

There's a set of skills you absolutely lose when you don't work in the hospital anymore. You get rusty at them. And these are different skills than what I use in the office. And it's good to have these skills, and understand how they make you think differently about the patient's condition. How to write a set of orders, managing intravenous fluids, or managing intravenous antibiotics as opposed to outpatient oral antibiotics, or managing the whole set of medications that we administer intravenously which is similar and complementary, but certainly different from what we use in the office. (Colin, family physician)

This raises a dilemma for PCPs. It may be equivalent or better from both an efficiency and quality-of-care perspective not to have office-based PCPs spend fragmented, intermittent time doing hospital medicine, and instead to trust this work to full-time doctors who work only in the hospital setting. However, at the same time, is anything lost that could affect the efficiency or quality of the office-based, ambulatory care PCPs provide? In essence, some of the PCPs were saying just this, that something important was lost, something only obtained by seeing and caring for patients at their sickest moments. While many PCPs identified specific advantages gained from hospital work for ambulatory care, such as greater familiarity with specialists in the area, exposure to new medical advances, cultivation of a different skill set, and experience treating advanced disease states, I got the sense that what PCPs lamented losing most was confidence from knowing that they had proven themselves as effective clinicians caring for patients at their worst.

This is a point not focused on enough in the debate about PCPs and hospital care. However, it is valid and relevant in considering the totality of the effects on PCPs of not doing hospital work. Much like any worker, PCPs derived a level of comfort by doing hospital work successfully that made them feel like better decision makers and clinicians on the outpatient side.

> Down there somewhere, there's still that feeling, "Well, if I'm not seeing sick patients in the hospital, then what good am I?" (Mark, internist)

The research on how patients feel about the use of hospitalists is sparse and inconclusive. A few studies have shown that patients are satisfied with having hospitalists care for them.[8] But it is unclear to what extent the patient samples included had regular primary care physicians, or if they based their feelings of satisfaction on a comparison between hospital care from a regular PCP versus that from a hospitalist. In addition, it is meaningful but only part of the story to ask patients or their families to comment on how satisfied they are with hospital care. That satisfaction is closely related to how effectively their clinical needs are taken care of when they are inpatients, and how quickly they leave the hospital. What is more difficult to tap into is how patients and their regular PCPs feel about their mutual relationship when the latter turns over hospital care to a strange physician, someone the patient has never met before.

A quarter of PCPs in the study, particularly the older ones who had long done hospital work, believed that its absence weakened the trust patients had in them and hurt continuity of care. The trust issue gnawed at them particularly. Trust was a commodity already made more difficult to obtain in a workday of fifteen-minute visits and assembly-line medicine. PCPs worried about how patients perceived them after having been through a hospital stay without ever hearing from their regular PCP.

> When you see your patients through a serious illness in the hospital, there's a tremendous bonding that occurs. They appreciate it so much. (Jane, family physician)
>
> .　.　.
>
> If it's something simple or a younger patient, it might be fine. But the sicker patient, the elderly patient, who still has that vision of, "Well you're my general doctor and you take care of everything," that's more problematic. Most of the elderly patients don't like it. They get good care, that's fine. But they want to see their doctor, who takes care of them every day, direct them through care. (Gary, internist)
>
> .　.　.

> Like I said, we hung onto our hospital care probably for longer than any other primary care group in the area. Only because we wanted to provide that service to our patients. And it's taken patients a while to adjust to it. They've gotten to know the hospitalists now a little bit. But I still get a lot of patients who come to me and say, "You know, Doc, five years ago when I had a heart attack you showed up at the ER door and I felt safe. And last month, when I had my heart attack I didn't feel safe with the guy who was there because I didn't know him, but I know you." It's unfortunate. (Francis, family physician)

Almost all PCPs felt that continuity of care was undermined when they did not care for their patients in the hospital. In their estimation it was undermined for two main reasons: the reality of a hospitalist taking care of a patient with whom they had no prior relationship, and the dangers of not having complete clinical information moving back and forth in a timely manner between PCP and hospitalist.

> When you've been the one caring for the patient, and then something serious happens and they go into the hospital, and now some physician who's never treated them before, or doesn't have all the information ready at their disposal, you can't help but think that hurts patient care in some way. (Rick, internist)
>
> .   .   .
>
> What the hospitalist model has done is remove the primary care physician from the hospital portion of care. And that's to the patient's loss. There is an advantage to continuity of care. And it's tougher for us to catch up with what's happened in the hospital when we have to go out and get records or discharge summaries as to what went on. (Colin, family physician)
>
> .   .   .
>
> The patient goes to the hospital, they want to see you, you want to see them, but you can't because you're stuck here in the office. They're disappointed, and you're disappointed. They come back to you, it's an even bigger nut to crack because you've got to go over everything that was done in the hospital, make sure you got all the medications straight, make sure you got all the testing done and follow up on it. And a lot of times you may not even have all the records you need, or you don't know if and what you might still be missing. (Sal, internist)

The off-loading of hospital work by PCPs is likely to continue. It is a necessary and strategic response by both hospitals and primary care offices to the reality of decreased hospital reimbursement and the increased complexity of hospital care. Hospitals prefer physicians who are on-site twenty-four hours a day to monitor, care for, and prepare for discharge inpatients for whom reimbursement is fixed to a set time period. PCPs are paid so little for seeing their patients in the hospital that they can generate better reimbursement doing ambulatory care visits in the office. Patients are so much sicker in the hospital now that there is a larger amount of clinical knowledge needed to manage their care, and physicians trained only to do hospital work have more of that knowledge and experience at their disposal. As a result, the field of hospital medicine, made up almost exclusively of physicians, is likely to grow, recruiting to its ranks many doctors who might otherwise become primary care physicians. From the twin perspectives of efficiency and quality of inpatient care, the health care system may do fine without PCPs as part of the hospital division of labor. There is sound logic to the notion that doing something a lot makes you more familiar with and better at it, and PCPs have less and less opportunity to do hospital medicine even if they wanted.

But the absence of PCPs from the hospital medicine scene can worsen negative dynamics already endemic to our health care system. First, it further fragments care for all patients in a system where it is already hard to know whom to trust. For sicker or elderly patients who may use the hospital more, it heightens the probability that things will be missed in their care, and that they will not have their care managed in a manner that is truly holistic and continuous.

It will also increase the level of cynicism some patients feel toward their doctors, regardless of specialty. This is because such cynicism is a direct outgrowth of a lack of regular contact with the same medical professional over time, a medical professional in whom patients place their faith to look out for them, especially at their most vulnerable. Do I personally care if my primary care physician takes care of me when I am in the hospital? Probably not. But I also presently do not have a PCP with whom I have built up a relationship over time. I have no complex chronic disease to manage, nor do I suffer from a serious health condition that puts me in the hospital at unexpected intervals. I also am familiar enough with how health care delivery works not to need detailed explanations for why things happen the way they do. Other types of patients, those who have different relationships with their physician, are in poorer health, or possess less knowledge about health care might be less inclined to accept that their PCP does not show up in the hospital to take care of them or hold their hand.

The absence of hospital work makes a primary care career instantly more appealing to young doctors who have lifestyle on their minds. But it also makes primary care medicine more routine in the process. Sacrificing hospital care completely will produce PCPs with a narrower skill and experience set to draw upon in the conduct of everyday office care. For increasingly sicker patients walking into the PCP's exam room each day, this cannot be a good thing. It will also further the declining prestige and value of primary care work, which may provide enough justification to keep salaries for primary care specialties on the flat trajectory they have experienced for sometime now.

More to the point, as a generation of older PCPs who did hospital care their entire career retires and gets replaced by doctors who have never done any hospital care outside of residency, the field ends up with practitioners that know their patients much less than they should. This reality brings with it a built-in potential for increased professional dissatisfaction that may trump the benefits gained from not having to get up at 5 A.M., be interrupted during a workday, or get home later in the evening. Being confined to a few office exam rooms for eight to ten hours a day may sound fine when you're thirty or thirty-five years old, if the pay is good and the hours are better.

But after twenty or so years, it could get pretty boring.

Chapter 5

The Routine and Nonroutine of Primary Care Work

There are strong perceptions that exist among medical students and residents that primary care work is too routine and less stimulating than specialty work. This view produces a psychological disincentive among these groups to choose a primary care specialty. To the extent primary care is imagined as lifestyle-friendly to students and residents in terms of having less intense, more flexible workdays, primary care may attract individuals looking for a healthier career choice while scaring away those who feel they deserve more given their training and personal sacrifices to become doctors. Central to this discussion is the nature of the work itself and how practicing PCPs see it.

This chapter examines primary care work in the early twenty-first century from the perspective of the individual PCP, and the types of patients and problems these professionals currently see on a regular basis. If today's primary care medicine does not involve the hospital or procedural work, and instead centers on ambulatory, office-based care for mostly acute care and chronic disease management, does it automatically become less intellectually gratifying to those physicians doing it? In addition, given the changes in the business model within which PCPs practice, it is relevant to explore whether or not a more transactional delivery system that makes physicians churn patients through more quickly and with less interaction affects the level of complexity in doing any type of primary care work. The types of patients visiting primary care offices also shape the degree of difficulty encountered in a given clinical situation. Thus, it is not only the work itself that matters, but the context within which that work is performed and how PCPs adapt that determine whether or not the practice of primary care is routine.

The Routine of Primary Care Work

PCPs take care of a lot of garden-variety medical conditions. Pediatricians have well-child visits and physical exams that make up over 20 percent of their work week.[1] These are visits where the work involved is predictable, standardized, and often performed on healthy patients. Few surprises or intellectual challenges may arise in the course of most healthy-child examinations. Similarly, almost 20 percent of a family doctor's and general internist's work week is taken up by general medical examinations.[2] While much of this adult preventive care is more complex than that done on children, due to sicker adults, a portion of it is routine. For all three primary care careers, acute care makes up over a third of total patient care, and routine chronic care another third.[3] A significant portion of this acute care may be for minor illness that carries with it no special challenge for the PCP.

For example, sinus and respiratory problems are not exciting medical conditions, at least after the first thousand or so. Within the typical eight-hour day of direct patient care, a PCP might see between 20 and 30 patients. Based on a five-day work week, that's 100 to 150 patient visits in a week. Out of those total patient visits, perhaps one-tenth will involve basic sinus and respiratory problems. That's probably conservative, because statistics show that anywhere from 15 to over 30 percent of all physician office visits in a given year involve respiratory symptoms alone.[4] Nonetheless, if 10 to 15 patients per week come with basic sinus and respiratory problems, that's 500 to 750 basic sinus and respiratory diagnoses treated over a fifty-week year. Based on a work career spanning thirty years, the PCP will diagnose and treat a total of between 15,000 and 22,500 basic sinus and respiratory problems. This care will be reproduced in a similar way each time: thousands of times of reciting "open your mouth wide," checking lungs, ears, and nasal passages, asking about the mucus color, maybe administering a strep test or drawing some blood, and then cutting a script for the same antibiotic over and over again.

All occupations, no matter how skilled or knowledge intensive, have work that is routine. Though this is work is less exciting to the person doing it, it is perhaps amenable to standardization in the techniques and thinking needed to execute it (thus done the same way repeatedly) and has fairly predictable outcomes over time. Having studied surgeons, emergency medicine physicians, and critical care physicians, three of the more "glamorous" specialties in terms of work variety, I have no doubt that every medical field has boring, repetitive work.

For example, how stimulating or unpredictable is the five-hundredth gall bladder removal or meniscus repair to a surgeon? Standardized treatment protocols exist for so many clinical situations now, including trauma care, that there is an inevitable element of the basic and mundane in all doctors' work. Despite television portrayals of medical work that consists of physicians arriving at diagnoses and treatments in often wildly original, hard-to-duplicate ways, the reality is that to work outside the appropriate standard of care in any field risks malpractice or chastising by peers, insurers, or one's employer. The reality of all medical work in the age of high-volume health care is to standardize and specialize labor as much as possible.

A friend had quadruple bypass surgery at a renowned heart center several years ago, and the entire work flow of presurgical, surgical, and postsurgical care was divvied up so that specific physicians had limited responsibilities in terms of what they did in that particular work flow. In short, each cardiologist and cardiac surgeon involved had a limited sphere of responsibility, and his or her job was to fulfill this responsibility reliably over and over again. This compartmentalized approach is often seen as leading to higher-quality care, since individual doctors can become masters over the knowledge and techniques it takes to execute specific steps in the context of a much more complex work process. But it also can turn any type of work, even highly technical, life-saving procedural work, into simpler, routine stuff to do.

Perhaps the key point is not that primary care contains any higher percentage of work that is considered boring or routine than other medical specialties, but that it contains work that society and the medical profession view as less meaningful than other specialties. For instance, research shows that when young doctors choose primary care careers, it is because they perceive it as more important than specialty care, and that others do not choose primary care because the work is viewed as less significant.[5] Societal trends in the types of physicians and medicine now seen on television, and glorified through the media, support the notion that while the country needs primary care, it does not want to hear about or be entertained by it. It is this type of negative perception that puts primary care in bad stead, and it means that primary care's routine work ends up at the bottom of the routine-work pecking order in medicine.

But is it really less meaningful as work? Is identifying a serious behavioral health issue in a patient for the first time and getting them treated less important than repairing a ligament in someone's knee? Is preventing a heart attack years in advance through the careful management of high blood pressure or cholesterol less meaningful than opening up an arterial blockage or installing a defibrillator in a person to avoid that same heart attack? Does preventing complications such as limb amputation or blindness in a diabetic patient through monitoring, care coordination, and education pale in comparison to the oncologist's work in administering chemotherapy to a cancer patient?

When the acute, urgent nature of many medical conditions is put aside for a moment, there is substance to the idea that primary care work may be the most meaningful medical work because, in theory, it can produce the all-around healthiest patient who avoids acute illness. Everyone wants the best cardiothoracic surgeon they can find if they need bypass surgery. But if individuals get to the point where they need bypass surgery, they likely did not interact meaningfully with the primary care system earlier in their lives to address the issues that now make surgery the only option. Thorough and regular physical exams, ongoing nutrition and lifestyle counseling, and chronic disease management may not sound sexy or high-tech enough in the twenty-first-century world. But they all work. And it is the PCP who knows how to do all of them best.

Through this lens, the bigger issue becomes less about objectively judging the "routine" or "nonroutine" nature of primary care work and more about the following: how the emerging realities of primary care practice, coupled with decisions made by PCPs to adapt to those realities, have changed the scope and substance of primary care work.

The Narrowing Scope of Primary Care Work

PCPs were uniform in their assessments of the direction in which primary care work was moving. In addition to the routine acute and preventive care that is traditionally a significant portion of the PCP's workday, primary care work now involved little or no hospital care, little emergency care, increased case management and care coordination responsibilities, fewer procedures done on patients, and a dramatically rising number of behavioral health issues to decipher and treat. For family physicians and general internists, larger numbers of patients now came into their exam room with multiple chronic diseases, and more of these patients were unhealthy. There were differences in how PCPs perceived these various changes.

Billy is a middle-aged general internist who conveyed brutal honesty in his perception of what existing realities had done to primary care work. He felt strongly that primary care medicine was more basic than ever. It was this conclusion that had moved him into a new kind of practice business model several years ago, which for him provided more profit and intellectual stimulation. This new model involved employing less costly nurse practitioners and physician assistants to see many of his patients, offsetting the decreased fee schedules to which his work was subject and the decrease over time in lucrative procedural work. Billy thought PCPs on the whole had a much easier workday now and that all the talk about how difficult it was had little basis in reality.

If there's one thing I can tell you about primary care and how it's changed over twenty years, it is that there is a lot less responsibility now than there used to be. A lot less burden on the practitioner, and that's why I can do so many things. The first burden is that I had to go to the hospital. If I was on the staff of two hospitals that meant each day I had to spend two to four hours doing rounds at these places, not to mention when you got called back to the hospitals for one of your patients. The second thing is physician assistants and nurse practitioners can do everything that a primary care doc can do right now. I've hired a bunch of NPs and PAs and when they run into something they don't know, they come to me for a consultation. I can run multiple offices and oversee everything and it works out fine. From the perspective of what a primary care internist does that an NP or PA can't do these days, the answer is nothing. Nothing. And so insurance companies are paying us less and less. And patients don't give a darn whether they see me with board certification or an NP. Doesn't matter. The fact is if they heard my name and good things attached to it, when they come to my office they don't care who they end up seeing. If I was a consumer, I wouldn't be that way. But the consumer is always right.

The specialists have to wake up at 5 A.M. and get to the hospital to get their procedures done so they can get to the office and see patients. Primary care docs don't do that. We have hospitalists taking care of our patients in the hospital, so we're not up in the middle of the night. We don't have to go to the hospital in the morning. We only book as many patients in a day as we want to see. We're not in urgent care anymore that much. Urgent care centers are all over the place now. So if we're not in urgent care, patients have appointments and they come to my office. And if a patient comes to my office without an appointment, I have a choice about whether or not I want to see them that day. It's different than before. Much different. (Billy, internist)

Colin, a family physician in his late fifties, was less blunt than Billy but still conveyed a similar feeling that primary care work had a smaller scope of responsibility now, which for him made it less exciting and satisfying. For many years, Colin had taught and worked in a family medicine residency program treating a poorer, sicker population. Colin focused on how family physicians had fewer procedures to do in their everyday work compared to ten or fifteen years ago.[6] This work had been ceded to specialists such as orthopedists, hospitalists, and general surgeons, and to new practice settings such as freestanding urgent care centers present in almost every larger community.

Anything that calls for procedural type activity, meaning a laceration, an injury, stepping on a nail, whatever, folks have gone from using their primary care physician to using their nearest specialist or urgent care center. That did not used to be the way it was. Our scope of work keeps decreasing. The amount and type of procedures we do has changed, and become a lot less. If we're looking at laceration repairs, for example, I still do them but we're doing a lot fewer. Splints and casts for straight up fractures, for an ankle, a level 1, 2, or 3 sprain, avulsion fractures, fractures of the metatarsal, things we normally would've taken care of—almost without fail the patient now goes off to the orthopedist for the splint and care during and after. Fewer people come in looking for us to treat things like straightforward fractures. They go right to the orthopedist without us even knowing. Especially if they have the type of insurance plan that lets them bypass us.

Normally, in family practice we would do uncomplicated cyst aspirations. Now, we'll send them to a general surgeon whether they're complicated or uncomplicated. Most family docs today wouldn't even think of doing a cyst aspiration. And these are fairly straightforward situations, when we know it's a cyst and it's just a matter of draining it, sending the fluid off to pathology for testing. Certainly, if you're looking at expenses, you add on significantly by changing where a procedure like this gets done. Send them to a surgeon, the surgeon does it, they do a follow-up—that costs more than us doing it. Since we do less hospital care, we do less newborn care. Family docs used to do things like circumcisions. We don't do that stuff anymore.

Also, what we call "lumps and bumps," excision of suspicious lesions, we don't do a lot of that anymore, either. Invariably, we'll go to plastics or a general surgeon to get it done for the patient. So, we pare down into fairly straight medicine, fairly straight peds.

Personally, I think primary care's a lot less interesting than it used to be. I understand in family medicine, for example, we're fairly broad. But doing these other things, like procedures and tending to things like simple bone breaks and fractures, made for more variety. You would end up having to switch hats several times during the day. Just being a case manager only, for example, is a lot less interesting than going ahead and doing some of the stuff you're now managing. And I know I can do that stuff as well as anyone else, and at lower cost to the entire system. So it's less fulfilling at the end of the day for me personally by not doing things like procedures myself. (Colin, family physician)

All PCPs in the study acknowledged that their scope of work had changed dramatically compared to the generalist practicing in 1970, or even the PCP in 1990. Many, like Colin, interpreted this change as a "narrowing" of their work, characterized by fewer unique tasks to do in the course of a given day and decreased complexity in the skill set needed to do the work that remained. Besides losing hospital medicine and most office-based procedures to physicians outside of primary care, PCPs did work with patients suffering from chronic disease that grew increasingly routine and standardized.

The application of clinical guidelines makes exam room work more predictable, can homogenize the PCP's view of patients in less than ideal ways, and narrows the zone of discretion PCPs employ during a clinical encounter. On the plus side, it increases the chance that patients with the same disease received similar, appropriate care.[7] But it forced PCPs within a limited amount of time to structure patient interactions in a way focused primarily on ensuring that the guideline "to dos" were done and the right boxes on the guideline template checked. To avoid full compliance with the guideline risked not being paid by insurers for the visit and violating standards of care that could get them sued later on. However, the trade-offs for this compliance were the reduced potential for new insights to be gained from the encounter and less of the physician's "art" in the practice of medicine. In a world of guidelines, the value of serendipity through treating each patient as a unique individual is not easily recognized.

PCPs also spoke of an important choice they faced with more complex patients which directly impacted their scope of work. This was the choice of whether and how quickly to refer a patient to a specialist. This is one of the most important decisions made at the primary care level. It involves an assessment by PCPs of their own ability to perform equal to or better than the specialist in diagnosing and treating the patient's condition in a timely manner. Many PCPs spoke of their increased tendency to refer patients with complicated or uncommon symptomatic presentations more quickly to the appropriate specialist. This finding showing the relationship between the perceived degree of difficulty in a clinical situation and PCP referral decisions has been observed elsewhere.[8] For quicker referral decisions, it reduced the variety in their work and the intellectual stimulation encountered in a typical workday. But it was clear that the pressure to achieve the production targets that earned revenue for the practice, in terms of set numbers of patient visits, forced some of them to refer more quickly than they would like.

You get back these abnormal tests. And there was a day I would get on the Internet or go through my medical textbooks, and open up the books and say "this is the problem" and read through it, and decide that this should be the next step in the workup, and get that information back and say, "OK, this is positive or negative," and go through that again and keep doing the "what's the next step, what's the next step." And now, the test is abnormal and I'm like, "Let's send them to the specialist." The specialist can do the workup. "This is abnormal, what do I do with it. Well, it's not on the top of my head." Send them to the specialist. And the shame is that because of my training, I am prepared to work patients up much more than the average primary care physician. I'm used to looking at these incidental findings and it's intellectually stimulating, to look things up and say, "OK, this is what's happening and this is the next step in ordering the scan or urine test or whatever's necessary." But now it's like, I say to myself, "I have thirty seconds to look at this test." So off they go to the specialist. And there is a time when you have to refer to the specialist. But there's a lot of things I know I can work up just given an extra ten minutes to mull things over, and contemplate what's good and bad. (Caitlyn, internist)

. . .

One of the things I miss that comes from being so pressed for time is that when the good, interesting case comes along, you've got five minutes to look at it and get out of the exam room. And you'd like to go back into your office, and read up on it, you'd like to do all that stuff, and you plan to do some of it, but more often than not, you do what you can and refer the patient out. Just because of the business need and press of patients in the day. (Mark, internist)

The pressures posed by patient visit demands on the scope of PCP work, and the subsequent choice made by PCPs to refer certain cases to specialists faster, was not limited to a specific type of PCP in the study. While one might expect certain groups such as younger PCPs to make referral decisions quicker, in part because their training and socialization within a specialty-dominated health care system provides less opportunity for diagnosing and treating complex patient conditions, later-career PCPs felt this pressure just as significantly. Here was the clear interplay between an evolving PCP work structure and individual physician adaptation to that new structure.

As the everyday impetus became seeing as many patients as possible, one specific adaptation by PCPs involved modifying their own expectations around how deeply into an "interesting" case they would go, and the precise time-point at which they were willing to give the patient over to a specialist for further care. They could see fewer patients in a day, refer out less quickly, and retain a greater portion of the stimulation and challenge deriving from playing the "detective" role in their work. In return, they would likely earn less compensation in the practice by seeing fewer patients than other PCPs, and potentially be viewed by colleagues as "less productive" given the lower comparable visit numbers. Or, they could modify their own rules used in assessing referral situations and in the process remain efficient in their workdays, mainly by referring patients to other doctors in the system more quickly.

The Complex Substance of Some Primary Care Work: Behavioral Medicine

A dramatic change in primary care practice that was not viewed as boring or routine were the increased numbers of children and adults with behavioral health issues. PCPs were uniform in stating how much of their overall workday was spent dealing with these issues.

> We do a tremendous amount of psychiatry here. Huge. And the insurance companies don't want to pay for that kind of stuff. But it's easy to get at if you want to. You can tell by people's affect. People will start crying in your office. I try to get them into some kind of counseling, try and find out why they're depressed, maybe their marriage is breaking up, or their son's a drug addict, the husband is dying of cancer. But there's long waiting lists for the mental health providers, the psychiatrists don't even do ongoing counseling anymore but instead just manage medications, and so you end up dealing a lot with it yourself. Just a tremendous amount of depression we see, every day, over and over. Dysfunctional childhoods, things like sexual abuse. And people never recover. (Rose, internist)

> · · ·

> The biggest change I've seen is the shifting of behavioral health and school-related issues into the pediatric setting, in part because there's not a lot of mental health providers for children at this point in time. I would say a third of my practice or more are kids with some behavioral issue. As a general pediatrician, there's always a layer of the behavioral, and that's OK. I'm not talking about how to talk with the parent about modeling behavior for the child, for example, or how to redirect behavior in a toddler. I'm not talking about the usual social and behavioral things.

But, if you read the statistics, one of every four kids is on some psychotropic med. And I wasn't trained to use or manage those meds. This is a real challenge for pediatricians right now. Even if you like doing it, trying to fit it into your day and figure out how to do it right, is a big challenge. (Maura, pediatrician)

. . .

The adolescents take a huge amount of time, and it can eat up a lot of your day if you're not careful. You have to see the adolescent with the parent, then see them alone, then bring the parent back in. The worst part of it is the social part. More and more of them have psychological or behavioral problems. A lot of kids who need counseling, and I just do not have the time nor do I get paid to do the counseling. So we end up shipping them out, but the counselors out in the community are getting fewer and fewer. They end up in our practice and we have to deal more directly with them, treating them. As the kids are getting pushed to grow up faster and faster, we're running into more issues with them. The nuclear families are basically falling apart, and the parents don't know what to do because they don't have their parents around to talk to about it. We end up being the prime resource for the parents, giving them advice, helping them figure out what to do. (Steven, pediatrician)

. . .

I have always said they should put Lexapro in the drinking water here in this town.[9] That's how many people I get walking through my door with some sort of depressive or anxiety disorder. (Mick, family physician)

The statistics are staggering in this regard. In the pediatric setting, behavioral health has by necessity become the purview of the general pediatrician. Shortages of child psychologists and psychiatrists in every community force pediatricians to get involved in the diagnosis and treatment of behavioral health problems. For example, one study using National Health Survey data found almost 6 million outpatient visits occurring between 1995 and 2002 by U.S. children between the ages of two and eighteen during which an antipsychotic medication was prescribed. Eighty percent of these visits occurred in physician offices, and almost one-third of the total prescriptions occurred in visits to pediatricians, family practitioners, emergency medicine physicians, and others who were not psychiatrists.[10] The number of antipsychotic prescriptions for children increased over 500 percent between 1995 and 2002.[11]

The National Survey of Children's Health has found that almost 10 percent of children ages three to seventeen are identified by their parents as having moderate or severe difficulties in one or more areas involving emotions, behavior, concentration, or ability to get along with others.[12] Almost 8 percent of children age six to seventeen in this same survey were found by their parents to have problems with social behaviors.[13] Finally, the parents of over one-third of children under the age of five expressed concerns about one or more of the following: behavior, getting along with others, the ability to do things for themselves, and preschool and school skills.[14]

In adult primary care, over a quarter of adult Americans suffer from a diagnosable mental disorder in a given year, with half of that group having two or more mental health diagnoses simultaneously.[15] Depression is the leading cause of illness in the United States for individuals ages fifteen to forty-four, and affects almost 7 percent of the general population.[16] Among diagnosed patients, 42 percent with clinical depression and 47 percent with generalized anxiety disorder (GAD) were first diagnosed by a primary care physician.[17] One recent study of National Health and Nutrition Examination survey data found that psychotropic medication use in the U.S. adult population almost doubled from 6 percent during 1988–1994 to 11 percent during 1999–2002. Significant increases in the use of antidepressants were seen among all adult age groups between the two time periods.[18]

The focus on behavioral health is a new part of the PCP's workday in the twenty-first century. Most PCPs liked the fact that behavioral health issues increased the variety in their clinical work. It presented greater complexity in decision making around both diagnosis and treatment that was seen as challenging and rewarding.

> I like this part of my job. Because when you help someone through a difficult time, they're really thankful, and it's really rewarding to you. I had a patient come to me a few weeks ago. She told me she couldn't even get out of bed in the morning, couldn't function. Well, I took her into an exam room right away and we talked for about forty-five minutes. And I got her to calm down and feel OK walking out of here. We came up with a plan and as far as I know, it's a week later and she's sticking to the plan. Now that feels good, knowing that you can provide that kind of assistance. (Dillon, pediatrician)
>
> . . .
>
> There are certain areas where I feel I have a bigger impact than others. One of those areas is behavioral medicine. I just saw a woman yesterday. Headaches, headaches, headaches. Horrible headaches. I questioned her a little bit further and she got all tearful and said, "I don't understand,

my life's good, why am I like this, why am I crying?" And after a thorough physical exam and history, and after talking her down a bit, I still did the medical work-up. But did I think the head CT I ordered on her would make her feel better? No. Do I think the fact that she's going to follow up with me, and talk more with me, and I'm trying to get her to a counselor, do I think those things matter more, that will make her feel better? Yes. And ultimately I feel like I connected with that patient, and you could see the relief spread across her face after she was able to talk to me about it. (Wilma, family physician)

. . .

I am stimulated by the psychosocial part. When I find out that I can help a person by altering the chemicals in their brain, or showing them the "why" of something, or helping get them to the right kind of therapy. My old partner, as soon as someone showed any signs of anything emotional that was overlaying their medical stuff, he sent them right off to a psychiatrist or psychologist. I find it very gratifying and interesting. My favorite story—I had a forty-year-old patient, father of two youngsters. I met him twice before. College-educated guy. He walks in and says, "I heard there's a medicine that can help people like me. I have an obsessive compulsive disorder and I'd like to start that medicine. I've known you for only two visits, but now I feel comfortable telling you this story." (Frank, internist)

Despite the internal reward felt by PCPs, there was little routine about much of this behavioral health work. One reason it was not routine was because few PCPs had much formal or extensive training to diagnose and treat these types of issues. Many spoke with trepidation about their competence to practice behavioral medicine.

I enjoy it but am forced to learn a lot on my own. If I am going to deal with it in my practice. Especially the medication management part. We don't get taught that stuff in medical school and residency. And I'm pretty comfortable now, after taking some continuing education courses and doing a lot of reading, with the moderate disorders like attention deficit-disorder and hyperactivity disorder. But when you start moving more into things like bipolar disorder, I get much less comfortable. Because the medication part is a lot more complex. (Dillon, pediatrician)

. . .

I was never trained to use the meds we put kids on these days, so it's a steep learning curve for me. I am never completely sure how much of this stuff we should be handling, or how prepared I am to take care of it.

But there's so much of it hitting you, you have no choice. You have to know your limits, and where your ability to understand or treat the problem ends. (Maura, pediatrician)

. . .

You know you have to do it, because it ends up being right there before you, but you find yourself always asking, "How comfortable am I with moving forward on this?" And I can tell you, in residency you don't learn how to handle behavioral diagnoses, other than seeing the real extreme cases of mental illness that end up presenting in an inpatient setting. And in an office setting, that's not what you're going to see. In family practice, compared to medicine, we probably get a little more exposure to it during our training. But I find now that it helps a lot to have access at key times to the input from a psychiatrist I can talk to, or I have to spend a lot of time on the Internet reading about stuff myself, and trying to make sense of it. (Peter, family physician)

No PCP in the study felt completely able to handle the full range of behavioral issues that might arise in a primary care setting. What made matters worse, besides the lack of training, was the existing structure of the primary care workday, in particular the reality of the fifteen-minute visit where many behavioral diagnoses first revealed themselves. This was the second element that made a PCP's behavioral medicine work move beyond the routine. The internal tension faced by some PCPs derived from balancing their own fears about "missing something" against the Pandora's box quality associated with exploring the patient's psychosocial state in a compressed time period. No PCP wanted to miss something that was important. But the reality of patients crowded up against each other in the daily schedule, and the fact that reimbursement for behavioral health care in primary care settings ranged from nonexistent to insufficient, made practicing behavioral medicine risky from a financial standpoint and work not easily standardized.

There are some insurance companies that won't even reimburse a primary care setting for treating patients with depression. Generally, the reimbursement models don't recognize the complexity of this kind of work, and if you uncover it in a visit where the patient is there for something else, which is usually the case, well, you get conflicted because you don't want to have to ask the patient to come back for the behavioral problem, but you also know that you won't be able to bill for it at that visit in a way that covers all the time you might spend with them. (Maura, pediatrician)

Why Primary Care Will Remain the Epicenter
of Behavioral Health Care

In the twenty-first century, the primary care exam room is the locus for patients to "open up" and reveal psychosocial issues affecting their health. It is the first-line triage point for mental health diagnoses. The reason why primary care settings remain front-and-center in this regard is threefold: they are the main access point into the health care system for almost everyone; limited numbers of psychiatrists and psychologists are available in many communities; and coverage in many health insurance plans for mental health consultations and treatment remains inadequate. With so much foot traffic coming through the primary care door, the more a PCP wants to ask and listen in a workday of twenty brief visits, the higher the likelihood some percentage of those visits reveal a behavioral diagnosis. In this way, any routine encounter can quickly grow complex and time consuming, making the workday unpredictable, stressful, but also exciting for the typical PCP.

All PCPs mentioned how "listening to the patient" during the exam room encounter was the critical ingredient in doing their jobs right, particularly when it came to spotting and diagnosing behavioral health issues. But listening takes time. Loretta is a family doctor who works in an urban-practice setting. She sees many patients in the course of a given day who present on the schedule as simple, short visits but, once in the exam room, present a range of problems that she must listen to, digest, and then act on in some way, turning the routine patient into one often needing much more.

> It's difficult in the time you have to deal with the psychosocial issues that patients have. I had a patient who came in with continuing ankle pain. Now she's had like four operations on her ankle and she's in for a fifteen-minute visit. And while I'm looking at the ankle and asking her some questions, she just says, "You know there's a lot of sites on the Internet devoted to suicide, did you know that?" And I'm like, "OK, well, that's fine but why would you be saying that?" And slowly she just starts to open up, telling me how bad she feels, how this is not the way she wanted to end up, not being able to do things with her grandchild because of the ankle problem, and having to go through all these surgeries and still not being better. That's not anything I could anticipate when I saw her on the schedule, but that's what ended up being the focus of the visit—her depression around the ankle and what it's done to her life. Those things happen a lot, and every situation's a little different and requires a little different approach. You can never assume that any

patient doesn't have something else they're hiding that they want to share with you. And you can never predict when and where it's going to reveal itself, which makes every time you go into that exam room a bit of an adventure.

Two days ago, I had a lady come in for a regular GYN checkup. And she talked to me about being sexually abused. And this was her first GYN, and she talked to me about why this was only her first GYN checkup. She had never had one before. What I had to do was talk to her about it for a while, ultimately refer her to a counselor, but during the procedure it was not just a simple GYN. I talked all the way through it so she was comfortable.

I saw a twelve-year-old today that's been refusing to get out of bed. And her mother doesn't think its physical, and I don't either. I think there's something going on at school. And we did blood work today. But she's going to have to come back and answer some questions, and we're probably going to have to get the school psychologist involved. Today, I must've had four or five patients who had physical complaints, but when I talked to them some more I felt that there was something more there. Depression. Or maybe that their life just stinks and they need someone to talk to about it. And a lot of times you get the first wind of it right when you're putting your hand on that doorknob to leave the room. (Loretta, family physician)

As I spoke with Loretta, I realized how much she seemed to want to know these things about her patients. Like other PCPs interviewed, her overt frustrations arising from when and how patients often presented their psychological issues to her, perhaps at the end of an already too long visit, or in a thinly veiled way that required her to dig into the conversation, belied a deeper commitment to helping individuals sort through their mental health issues. Like other PCPs, she chided a health care system that would not recognize her important role as patient advocate and first diagnostician of behavioral disorders. She felt isolated in her everyday work because of this feeling, and it appeared to lessen her job satisfaction.

The typical primary care practice, regardless of geographic location, deals with behavioral health issues in larger quantities than ever before. Although primary care work generally is narrowing in its scope, this aspect of it adds substance and complexity to the PCP's workday. PCPs have difficulty practicing behavioral medicine because of the current primary care business model and limited training of PCPs in behavioral medicine. It also makes behavioral medicine a reactive rather than proactive endeavor on the part of PCPs, given the intense competition among different symptoms and complaints for the limited time available to each patient during his or her exam room visit.

PCPs already have much to do for patients in a visit. They must consider their chief complaints, acquire relevant patient history, conduct a brief physical exam, administer relevant clinical guideline requirements, enter information into an electronic health record or paper chart, check the need for refilling prescriptions, and have some basic level of conversation with patients about their life situations. By themselves, none of these activities are overwhelming for a competent PCP. However, pushed into a fifteen-minute encounter they combine to challenge the PCP's ability to deliver quality care in every instance.

Primary care physicians have chosen to give up hospital medicine. They also now perform few procedures in their offices. These changes have decreased the variety in their workday and enhanced the capacity to assume clinical work that may involve less complex chronic disease management through the application of standardized guidelines and simpler forms of acute care. But the non-routine aspects of primary care work remain significant still, despite the absence of this other work, because the individuals visiting primary care today are sicker and bigger mysteries to PCPs, and because the prevalence of behavioral disorders has grown.

PCPs can explore these mysteries and their accompanying diagnoses given time, proper reimbursement, and appropriate skill development. But without these ingredients, the reality is less routine work that frustrates PCPs and complicates their day. And if listening to and asking questions of patients are the pathways to doing more of this work, logic dictates that some PCPs will behave in the exam room in ways that limit the conversation, stick close to the guideline if there is one, and make the patient's chief complaint the only legitimate clinical focus.

Part II

The People Doing Primary Care Work

Chapter 6

Younger and Older Physicians in Primary Care

If there is one thing on the minds of many young and aspiring physicians in the early twenty-first century, it is "lifestyle".

> People go into a lot of specialties now, not just primary care, to have a better lifestyle. I have a friend who is in a radiology residency, and she clearly said it was because she wanted to be home with her kids at the same time every afternoon. And I said to her, "Won't you get bored sitting in a dark room all day?" And she said, "Yeah, probably, but I'll be home in the afternoons with my kids." So, it's a trade-off for her. (Stephanie, first-year resident, family physician)

> . . .

> I like medicine a lot. But I don't want to do what my father did, who was a pediatrician, working all hours of the week, coming home usually after we all ate supper, being there late at night and on weekends for patients. I want to have some semblance of a normal life. (Tom, thirties, internist and pediatrician)

> . . .

> I want to be happy not just as a doctor, but also as a person. I value other things in my life and want to be able to pursue those things. (Harry, thirties, internist)

> . . .

> I won't be able to do crazy-hour work weeks, or work eighty hours a week. That's just not an option for me. (Lance, second-year medical student)

> . . .

My practice partner works three and half days per week, because he wants to do other things and his wife is a professional, so he can do that. A lot of us are interested in having a better lifestyle and using the other resources available like urgent care centers and hospitalists, so we're not encumbered with our practice twenty-four hours a day, seven days a week. And, overall, I think it's good. If you're burned out at the end of every day, you can't do that well. (Gary, thirties, internist)

Lifestyle is now a critical factor determining which specialties medical students choose. A 2003 study in *Journal of the American Medical Association* found for 100,000 medical students graduating each year over a seven-year period by far the largest explanatory factor for specialty choice was "controllable lifestyle." This factor increased in importance among senior classes over the span of the study. It was also cited by students five times more frequently as a driving factor for specialty choice than "average income."[1] In the early twenty-first century, the misconception may be that most medical students become certain types of physicians only "for the money." That may true for a small segment of medical students, especially those with large debts. But there is now an overt desire on the part of both male and female medical students and residents to get paid well and be in a specialty that has bounded hours, predictable workloads, and enough time off. In short, many fledgling doctors want to have it all.

There's a perception of what the softest specialties are that you can get the biggest paychecks out of while still having a great lifestyle, like ophthalmology and dermatology. But those are also the hardest specialties to get into right now, for exactly that reason. (Lance, second-year medical student)

Daniel is a third-year medical student in his late twenties who has already worked several jobs before coming to medical school. He is coldly calculative in his assessment of the types of medical careers in which he and, in his opinion, other student colleagues are interested.

As time goes on, students change and they have different expectations. I think we're willing to put up with a little bit less now, in terms of the demands that becoming a doctor places on you. I've got a short list of things I'm really interested in, and a few things I'm not interested in. Not so much because the jobs themselves are not interesting or that I don't think I couldn't make a positive difference doing these specialties. But rather because I think as a career, not only dealing with patients but with all the other intangibles and tangibles like lifestyle, pay scale, difficulties dealing with insurance reimbursements, difficulties dealing with other doctors and ancillary staff, those careers are much less attractive.

So the short list of those specialties that look really good, I mean, you just have to look at the graduating classes and see where the most competitive applicants are going towards. And those are the most attractive careers. Because by and large medical students aren't dumb. They tend to gravitate towards specialties where they'll have the greatest return on their investment, not just the money but other things too. So anesthesiology, radiology, dermatology are all popular. Even pathology is becoming popular. Because it's minimal patient contact, the hours are very predictable, and the reimbursement is actually really, really good.

Primary care is becoming less and less attractive as time goes on. As a medical student, even before I went to medical school, I knew that. It's getting to the point where if I had thought when I went into medical school that I would have had to be a primary care doctor, I don't think I would've gone to medical school. Because although primary care is rewarding, all the other things that come with having a career make the trade-off not worth it. You understand that we have four years of undergraduate, four years of medical school, a minimum of three years of residency, oftentimes we're graduating with $200,000 or $300,000 of debt. I have to think of how am I going to pay this back and how am I going to have a decent quality of life for my wife and kids.

I like emergency medicine. It's kind of like primary care for a certain segment of the population. But you also get to see a wide variety of issues that people come in with, it's shift work, which is really nice, you can predict when you will go to work, when you're going to leave work. And being able to predict when you're not going to be working is something. I don't think people really understand the importance of that. When I was in my information technology job, network engineering, there were periods of time when I would be working on a project and be called at odd hours, because there would be a network installation and there might be problems. So I would get called at nine or midnight or three in the morning, and I would have to instantly deal with that issue. I know I won't have that with something like emergency medicine. (Daniel, third-year medical student)

For the field of primary care, it is hard to know which came first: PCPs interested more in their work as a job with defined work hours and boundaries, or the time-pressured, hectic everyday workload of PCPs that strain their willingness to view a medical career as something more than a well-paying, rewarding but far from 24/7 professional endeavor. There was strong evidence in this study that younger PCPs view their work as "a decent job" and less a calling, in large part because of the lifestyle benefits it offers.

That existing PCPs like the lifestyle associated with their primary care jobs might surprise medical students and residents who tend to perceive a primary care work career as too hectic, too diverse and overwhelming to do right on a day-in, day-out basis, and the pay too low commensurate with the demands.[2] In fact, some residents and students in the study who had not chosen general primary care as their career focus, or did not intend to, felt similarly. Daniel is one of those individuals. Such sentiment is rooted in the negative mythology around primary care that gets propagated within the medical training setting. For example, students and residents rotate through primary care practice environments where they often see too many harried and dissatisfied primary care doctors and a disproportionate number of sick, high-maintenance patients.

For individuals already in primary care, these negative perceptions of the career were present only in sporadic instances. This divergence between those doing the work and those not might be explained in one of two ways: once they are working, practicing PCPs adapt to the realities of primary care in a way that allows them to focus on the positive aspects of the job, in particular the lifestyle advantages (the "it's not as bad as I thought it would be" rationale), or most individuals who self-select into primary care fields already believe that primary care offers rewards that outweigh any potential negative realities around workload, pay, or job variety (the "I know what I'm getting into and am OK with it" rationale). These rationales are little different from ones maintained by other workers in society. Both the automobile assembly line worker and the convenience store cashier deal in trade-offs and rationalizations to equal degrees. In the present study, it appeared that a mix of both was at work in the younger PCP cohort.

Primary Care as a Decent Job

Despite the demands and pressures placed on PCPs in a typical workday, from seeing set numbers of patients in limited time frames to administrative demands and challenging cases, younger PCPs were largely satisfied in their jobs and felt that they had made the appropriate career choice. Of course, the cynic might counter with recent national survey data that show almost two-thirds of PCPs, regardless of age, stating they would not choose primary care again if given the choice.[3] However, as these and other surveys indicate,[4] PCP dissatisfaction with their work and practice environment appears more endemic among older PCPs, perhaps those trained and reared in a specialty-focused, less-corporatized health care environment not hostile to primary care.[5]

The assessment of primary care as a "decent job" derived from a combination of perceptions these individuals expressed about their work: there was an adequate level of stimulation and variety overall; the hours were predictable and not overwhelming, particularly for employees of a larger practice; and the pay, while less than other medical specialties, still sat well above the societal mean for all occupations and appeared fair given the greater flexibility and limitations in total work hours that were possible in some job arrangements. These perceptions were consistent across almost all younger PCPs. They appeared to mitigate the deleterious effects of a workday that could at times be routine, overly bureaucratic, hectic, and unpredictable.

Paul is a family physician in his early thirties. He is typical of many young PCPs interviewed as part of the study. He comes across as a pragmatist who sees primary care as a good fit for his skills and desires. He has structured his work career in a manner that allows him to work part time in a large primary care practice, and also to serve as a preceptor in a family practice residency program. Paul's wife is also a doctor. They have an infant and expect to have more children. At this early point in his career, Paul is content with the career choices he has made. For him, primary care is rewarding, in part because he maintains the above perceptions.

> I like everything in medicine. When I was on OB, I wanted to be an OB/GYN, when I was on pediatrics, I wanted to be a pediatrician. Everything interested me. I think what happened to me was that when I was going through my rotations in medical school I said, "I don't want to be in a room just reading films," or "I don't want to be just looking at the heart." I found that I kind of loved it all, and wanted to encompass as much as I could, so primary care fit. And in this job, I get to see a little bit of everything. Yes, I'll have lots of patients with diabetes or hypertension that need to be managed. But I'll also get to deal with women's health issues, which I love to do. I get to see kids and adolescents and see their unique problems. I have all the behavioral health stuff which is challenging.
>
> I remember when I was in medical school talking with other students about family medicine in comparison to, say, dermatology or radiology

or cardiology. And they said, "But you're going to be a jack of all trades and master of nothing, that would really bother me." For me, it didn't. If anything, I feel like it has grounded me a little bit. You don't know it all. You have to feel comfortable with what you do know. And when you're not comfortable with things you don't know, that's when you have to refer out. But the intimidation aspect can be big, because in primary care there's a big scope of work you have to cover. Here it works out for me because I have some older, more experienced docs that I can consult with, and we've got a nurse practitioner. If you have a group you feel comfortable, you can kind of feed off each other, and say "what do you think about this." That's nice. Being part of a larger group gives you that comfort level to be able to deal with the variety you see in your work. Solo practice would scare the heck out of me. Not just because I don't want to deal with the whole business side of things, but just because I wouldn't have that team with me everyday I could talk to.

Some of it's individualized. Some medical students don't want to have all that variety, aren't comfortable with knowing less about more. So they'll go into a narrower specialty where they can become the experts over that smaller amount of material. Me? I can't imagine not having the variety. And the money aspect of this whole thing to me is a bit overblown. You know, that all these people aren't going into primary care because the money isn't enough, especially if they have a lot of debt. But I have loans, so does my wife who's a pediatrician. And your school loans now are at such a rate where the interest is small, there are consolidation loans, there's ways you can do it. Me and my wife were paying back ours while we were still in residency. Some of it is what your expectations are, how you want to live. For us, the money's not an issue. Our jobs pay well enough.

Call here is about once a week, and every fifth weekend. We have a hospitalist service so if a patient goes to the hospital, we don't have to deal with that. The call involves having a pager. And on the weekend when you're on call, you come to the office on that Saturday morning and see patients for a few hours. I usually get home at six or six-thirty every night. If I need to finish up any notes or check on labs or anything, with the electronic record I can do that at home, just directly sign onto the system.

I'm still not really sure what I want to be when I grow up, but right now I am enjoying what I'm doing. It's challenging, but that's what it's supposed to be. (Paul, thirties, family physician)

Like Paul, other young PCPs, including all of those who worked full time, felt that their everyday work lives were manageable, and that the lifestyle benefits offered by primary care were tangible.

> I think I have a relatively easy lifestyle, easier than I thought I would ever have. I'm not on call very often. I have paperwork, but I can take some of it home to finish it if I need to. We probably could be reimbursed a little higher, but it's not bad. We all have loans we have to pay back. But we're still on the top of the income ladder, even if we don't realize it. I like where I work. I like my hours. No amount of money could make up for the time I like to spend with my family. It's all in what you make of it. (Lou, thirties, internist and pediatrician)

The word "lifestyle" is talked about so much as a motivating factor for young doctors today that it is difficult to understand whether it means the same thing for everyone. Younger PCPs in my study had a similar definition in mind, one that involved an equal mixture of "flexibility" and "predictability." Flexibility was defined as the freedom to move around jobs, work hours, and organizations.

> Family medicine is kind in terms of setting up your schedule the way you want it to be. That's one of the reasons why I work three different jobs. It keeps me from burning out in any one area, and it allows me the flexibility and excitement of different things every day. I work in this office a few days a week, at the local urgent care center a day a week, and I teach in a residency program a half day per week. I'm extremely marketable, I know that. Could I go to the Midwest or even another part of the state and make a lot more? Absolutely. But my family is here and this is where I grew up, and I like being around here. And I love keeping some variety in my workweek. (Wilma, thirties, family physician)

> . . .

> I like the ability to work in a couple different settings. That keeps it interesting. And at least early in my career, I want to be able to move around a little, to see what I might really like to do later on. (Paul, thirties, family physician)

Compared to older PCPs, more of the younger ones defined flexibility as working part time, three or four days per week as opposed to a normal Monday through Friday work schedule. This type of flexibility was particularly important to women with young children. A recent national survey of physicians found that 20 percent of both male and female physicians work part time, a trend that continues to increase.[6] For younger women, the ability to work part time can be important in helping to fulfill their goals as mothers who can spend meaningful time with their children. This same national survey showed that the overwhelming reason women physicians cite in working part time is to fulfill family responsibilities.[7] But flexibility was also important to male PCPs and female PCPs who did not yet have children. Almost half of PCPs under the age of forty who were interviewed in the study worked less than full time, which was defined as thirty-five to forty hours of direct patient care per week.

The Predictability of Today's Primary Care

The younger group also defined lifestyle in terms of predictability. Predictability, or the ability to know clearly the boundaries of the workday, was important to all of the younger PCPs in the study. When asked, this group was detailed in identifying the time they came into the office each day, when they left each night, and when, if at all, they did work in the evenings at home. Their description of the workday as a bounded nine- or ten-hour event, clearly separate from nonwork time, was different from that of older PCPs, who talked more loosely of when their typical days began and ended. Younger PCPs valued this regimented aspect to their careers because it made it clear to themselves and others that there was always a distinction between career and personal time.

> I think it's crucial to try and separate work from home. Even if that means on the way home each night, when I leave at 6 or so, I have to roll up the windows and turn the radio up a little louder, just to decompress and get the day out of my head, that's what I'll do. Then when I get home, we might talk about work for five or ten minutes at the dinner table, but that's it. (Harry, thirties, internist)

Almost all of the younger PCPs did some work after hours at home. This was due to the availability of an electronic medical record (EMR) system that enabled them to input clinical notes or check test results at any hour of the day.

> A lot of times, I'll bring some stuff home with me to work on. But I usually do it late at night, after I've had time to spend with my family, or see my child for awhile, and it's not that big a deal. If I don't have any catch-up to do, I don't do any work at night. (Lou, thirties, internist and pediatrician)

Like other jobs, information technology provided a virtual workplace where younger PCPs and their older cohorts could complete the administrative requirements of their jobs and get ready for the next day's patient schedule. In this way, EMR technology increased the predictability favored by younger PCPs by allowing them to limit surprises for the following day of visits. For younger PCPs this added work, outside of normal work hours, was stable in terms of content and time requirement. They talked more positively than older PCPs about how the availability of an EMR facilitated completion of the day's nonclinical demands at a time and place of the PCP's choosing. For some, this meant working an hour or two at 8 or 9 P.M., while for others it was work done as late as 11 P.M. or midnight.

Younger PCPs were not blind to the fact that the real predictability afforded by a primary care job came from the reduced scope of work in the job itself, and from being part of larger practices where after-hours work such as call could be distributed among bigger groups of doctors. This has already been touched upon but bears repeating here because it suggests a key paradox that speaks to the future trajectory of the primary care field. This paradox is the enhanced lifestyle that results for individual PCPs from a continued narrowing of primary care work and responsibilities.

For example, by no longer caring for patients in the hospital, there was less likelihood of events occurring during the workday that might delay PCPs in completing their visit schedules. As a result, the end of the daily schedule could be forecasted with greater certainty. There were also no calls at night from hospital emergency rooms, for example seeking approval for an admission from the PCP. There was no morning ritual wherein younger PCPs had to go early to the hospital and review their patients' status from the night before, which could delay when the normal office visit schedule began.

> I don't have to rush out of the house in the morning. I go straight into the office and since my patients don't start coming in until eight or eight-thirty, I can choose when I leave, or if I want to go in a little early to do some paperwork. But I know when that first patient is due in, so it's great in that regard. (Harry, thirties, internist)

Similarly, the movement in primary care work away from doing procedures on patients and accommodating acutely urgent visits in a typical patient schedule also increased the predictability of the workday. Procedures like colonoscopies, wound debridement and stitching, and casting or splinting contained greater time delays and uncertainty that could undermine a set office visit schedule. Having too many patients with urgent situations that arrived unannounced into the practice also undermined work-day predictability. The rise of urgent care centers and increased preferences of patients to go directly to specialists such as orthopedists reduced the work variety in a PCP's workday, but at the same time made it manageable. For younger PCPs who had never experienced years of episodes where the rewards and satisfaction from doing hospital work, procedures, or addressing a patient's emergency condition could produce satisfying memories, it was their ability to forecast the day's work with precision that defined their feelings of satisfaction.

Greater predictability also resulted from reduced call schedules associated with the larger practice settings where PCPs worked. Most of the younger and older PCPs in the study were on call perhaps one or two nights every week or every other week, with weekend call coverage often one weekend or less each month. This call schedule was a significant departure from the smaller primary care practices of the 1960s or 1970s, where one or two doctors might be on call every night or every other night. In addition, because of the absence of hospital medicine, much of this call responsibility involved lower-level interactions with patients who needed only a prescription refilled or a question answered. Anything that involved a potential hospital admission or emergency department visit, that is, anything too complex or acute, initially passed through PCPs but then went to the hospitalists taking care of the PCP's patients once an admission or emergency room visit had occurred.

Younger PCPs' Satisfaction with Their Compensation

Where compensation was concerned, younger PCPs admitted primary care jobs paid less, but with few exceptions were not put off by this reality.

> I do OK with my salary. I don't make as much as cardiologists or surgeons, but compared to the rest of society I earn a pretty good living. (Lou, thirties, internist and pediatrician)

Some of the younger group claimed to have lower debt burdens than their colleagues, and admitted that this was part of what enabled them to choose primary care as a career in the first place. They believed that primary care was a less appealing option for other student colleagues because of greater educational debt.

> I went to a state school for my medical training. So I didn't have hundreds of thousands of dollars of debt. So it probably was easier for me to pick primary care. I understand people who come out of medical schools with the equivalent of my mortgage on my house not ever ending up in primary care. (Tom, thirties, internist and pediatrician)

Many of the younger PCPs interviewed did have significant debt burdens, $100,000 to $200,000 in loans. While most expressed anxiety about their ability to pay back this debt with their existing salaries, they were satisfied with their pay. This raises an interesting question: When so many people criticize a primary care career because of lower salaries compared to other specialties, why is it that younger PCPs might not be as concerned about their compensation?

An obvious answer comes from the prior discussion of primary care as a decent job. Younger PCPs make trade-offs that include less pay for what they perceive as a better physician lifestyle. This may explain why the younger group emphasizes attributes such as predictability, flexibility, and time off as the key things they enjoy and desire in their careers. They may still owe a lot of money, but if the ability to move around jobs or go home unhindered at five or six each night is of utmost importance, the anxiety over debt becomes a lower priority, especially if they are single or without children. However, this does not tell the entire story. After all, specialties that pay much higher salaries such as radiology and dermatology also have predictable hours and enhanced lifestyles. But these other specialties are more competitive to enter relative to the welcoming arms of primary care, and may attract individuals with different personalities and talents than those entering primary care.

A second possible answer to why young PCPs appear satisfied with their compensation is the reality that younger PCPs are likely to be part of dual-income marriages so that, when taking into account the entire family income, lower PCP compensation is offset by a spouse's compensation in either medicine or some other career. This was the situation with Paul, the young family physician, and other young PCPs in the study. It is a national trend for physicians. A 1999 study of over 1,200 physicians who graduated from medical school between 1980 and 1990 found that almost one-fourth of male and one-half of female physicians were married to other doctors. Among women physicians, who go into primary care in greater numbers, over 90 percent of spouses in the same study worked outside the home.[8] As a result, the need to generate a single, high-paying salary is less critical. Theoretically, this would allow younger PCPs to view compensation differently, as only one component of an overall set of career expectations.

Finally, the compensation issue is confounded presently by the stark reality that primary care physicians are in high demand in the United States.[9] Many young PCPs may be more satisfied with their compensation because they are earning more than they thought they would, and because their marketability allows them to negotiate higher than average salaries. Over the past few years, salaries for general internists and family physicians have been on the rise. One national survey shows average salary increases of 19 percent and 9 percent between 2006 and 2008 for family practice and general internal medicine, respectively, after years of flat or declining trends.[10] This same survey also shows that family medicine and general internal medicine represented the largest number of physician search assignments requested by employers compared to all other medical specialties in a recent one-year period.[11] In addition, job searches for pediatricians increased 50 percent over a recent three-year period.[12]

Older PCPs in the study who functioned as medical directors and recruiters for their own practices felt strongly that it was a seller's market for primary care jobs at present, and that young PCPs knew it. They talked about the difficulty of getting some young PCPs to accept full-time jobs, as well as their own need to be aware of the array of benefits that young PCPs value.

> We lost two or three good young candidates about a year ago, because they went to other practices in the community that already had a hospitalist group working for them. Because these young docs didn't want to do hospital medicine. So, that was another reason why we switched over and gave our inpatient work to hospitalists. But we try and make the work environment one where young doctors want to stay for awhile. Because we don't want them cycling through for a year and then leaving. And more of them seem to want defined hours, they ask about how much call they will have, they don't want to do hospital medicine, and they want a certain pay level to start with. (Larry, internist and medical director)

Medical Training as a Primary Care Turn-off among Young Doctors

To believe young, aspiring doctors, medical training pays little attention to primary care. Add to this the general experience of becoming a physician now, from the hypercompetitiveness involved in getting into medical school to the mountains of financial debt many students incur, and there are nothing but disincentives for choosing a primary care career. Every young PCP, student, and resident interviewed implied that the choice to go into primary care was a courageous one, given a host of normative and financial pressures in medical training that pushed students and residents toward nonprimary care careers.

Anecdotally and in the literature, no issue is cited more frequently for the demise of primary care as a viable career choice than the issue of money. Because the typical medical school debt is over $100,000, not counting debt students may also have from their undergraduate education, and primary care salaries lag significantly behind what can be earned in other specialties, it is presumed that most students never think seriously about going into primary care.

> When you become a doctor now, you start out when you're thirty, and you basically have two mortgages hanging over your head. One for your house and one for your education. And you really feel like you're going to end up living paycheck to paycheck unless you go into some higher paying specialty. (Gary, thirties, internist)
>
> . . .
>
> To go out and do your cardiology fellowship and then start a job at $250,000 per year, versus $110,000 as a primary care doctor, that's a huge difference. And if you're on the hook for $200,000 or more in debt, you almost have to choose a better-paying specialty or else that debt is going to saddle you for a long time. You're going to pay that debt down a lot faster being a cardiologist than a primary care physician. End of story. In both my medical school and through residency, I saw people who might have considered primary care a lot more seriously if they didn't owe so much money. Instead, they went on to residencies like anesthesia or radiology, where after residency you are going to make double what you make in primary care. (Lou, thirties, internist and pediatrician)
>
> . . .
>
> If I was going to go into any sort of primary care field, it would be pediatrics. But I'm discouraged by what my financial situation is going to be when I graduate. All of my money for medical school is loans, which is about $60,000 a year. So, I'm going to graduate with about a quarter of a million dollars of debt. And it'll be tough to even pay off the interest on that during residency. So, we're talking upwards of $300,000 or more by the time I finish residency. At that point, salary makes a pretty big difference. Especially if you're a pediatrician making a $110,000 when you can make double or triple that going into a subspecialty. (Lance, second-year medical student)
>
> . . .
>
> It's such a pervasive notion among medical students. The thought of coming out with $100,000 or more of debt. And you look at the pay discrepancy between a primary care physician and pediatric cardiologist or cardiac surgeon, it's ridiculous. My uncle is an orthopedic surgeon and does spinal reconstruction, and makes $1 million a year. And he complains if he makes $700,000 or $800,000 in a given year. Part of it

is also that I've worked hard to get here and I deserve to be able to take a decent vacation every year, take some time off, and not feel like I'm scrambling to pay my bills like somebody working at McDonald's. And that's a real concern. Part of it is premature. You're not paying those loans back yet. You don't know what it's going to be like. But when you sign a promissory note for another $75,000, it scares the daylights out of you. (Daniel, third-year medical student)

Every medical student and resident mentioned the issue of debt when discussing the viability of a primary care career. In comparison to primary care, there are other specialties that provide both monetary and lifestyle rewards. Average salaries for jobs in radiology, emergency medicine, and anesthesiology, other "pro-lifestyle" specialties, are anywhere from 50 to over 100 percent higher than salaries in family practice or general internal medicine.[13]

But money and the need to pay back educational debt was only one source of ambivalence toward primary care among students and residents still completing their medical training. And as we saw among young PCPs, money was not the driving factor for career satisfaction. Another source for primary-care career discouragement in the medical training setting was the perception among medical students, medical school faculty, and residency programs that choosing primary care was a suboptimal choice, a career "consolation prize" that should only be considered when other options were not available.

A lot of my classmates feel like going into primary care would be settling for something less than they deserve, given how a lot of them had to fight to even get into medical school. There's also a connotation that primary care, especially pediatrics and family practice, is the "easy way out." And a lot of students think, "Well, why should I take the easy way out when I've had to work so hard just to be here?" (Molly, second-year medical student)

. . .

You definitely get a sense in med school that the smart kids, the ones doing the best, are not going to go into primary care, and shouldn't, and the kids in the middle or lower end of the pack are the future primary care doctors. It's sort of seen like if you're smart enough, you owe it to yourself to go into something other than primary care. It's funny, it's like, if you do well on a test, someone says to you, "Oh, but I thought you wanted to go into primary care?" I think everyone I know in med school recognizes there needs to be more primary care doctors. But a lot of them view it as the consolation prize. They say, "Yeah, there needs to be more of them but as long as I don't have to do it." (Zack, second-year medical student)

. . .

I think a lot of us view primary care as something beneath us, not as exciting as specialty care. I probably have the perception that it's more taking care of sick people who have basic chronic diseases like diabetes or heart disease. Not the interesting kind of sick but more the run-of-the-mill kind of sick. And, at this point in my career, I feel like I want to be involved in dealing with the interesting kind of sick. That leaves me thinking that even if I did primary care, I wouldn't want to just go out into some suburban practice and set up shop, but instead work in an inner city clinic or some really underserved area where I am going to see a wider variety of things, and be able to take care of more things because there won't be a lot of other specialists and people around to help. (Ben, first-year medical student)

Part of this negative view involved how some students saw the work involved in primary care.

I think a lot of medical students see primary care today as too routine and not on the cutting edge compared to other specialties, so they won't go into it. (Harry, internist)

. . .

Even if you pretended that none of the money stuff mattered for a second, medicine is so specialty oriented right now that if you get any patient with a serious medical condition, you end up referring them to a specialist anyway. You're sort of like a triage nurse as a primary care physician. That's kind of a turn-off. Some people see the upside of primary care as you get to see and treat a patient from when they're young to when they're old, you get to see whole families and they get to know you as their doctor. And that's true, and I think students realize that you get some more continuation of care you can't get in other specialties. But what I hear most often is the perception that primary care docs are this sort of triage person that sends patients off to specialists most of the time. (Lance, second-year medical student)

Part of the problem, in the opinion of study participants, lies in how medical schools structure their curricula. The first two years of training is classroom based, and most schools organize this pedagogy around organ systems (for example, nervous system, vascular system) or different pathologies (for example, cancer, heart disease). Basic science is at the core of first-year training.

Second-year training often emphasizes complex, interesting cases that illuminate specific disease processes. An increasing portion of training now centers on smaller group discussions and case studies.[14] A cursory review of several medical schools' initial two-year curricula shows little or no formal training focused on the clinical aspects of "generalist medicine" or "preventive medicine" or "primary care."[15]

Topics such as prevention and integrated care may be compressed into a student elective or two during this time, but largely remains peripheral to the emphasis on compartmentalized clinical systems.[16] Medical schools all have some form of clinical skills or practice course, but how much such a course is taught by primary care as opposed to specialist physicians is an open question. Students interviewed from two different medical schools felt that their first two years of medical school were characterized overall by high exposure to specialists and low exposure to primary care physicians, which did not help promote an interest in generalist medicine.

> A lot of the curriculum in medical school isn't based around primary care. It's more based around specialty care. It's always like, "Well when you have this case and you're the specialist in this scenario you deal with it this way." I don't think there's enough emphasis placed on original signs that you might notice as a primary care physician. I feel like medical school is always talking about "the rare case this" or "the rare case that," and it's always "the primary care physician screwed up and couldn't find it for ten years, and then the specialist finally found it after all this time." (Zack, second-year medical student)

. . .

> I don't think there's anything malicious, but our curriculum is organized around different themes throughout the year, and that theme leader is usually a specialist in that field. So we're exposed to a very large number of specialists and as far as primary care physicians, I can maybe think of only two or three we've been exposed to thus far, that have actually interacted with us. In the first year, the themes are broken down into organ systems, cardiovascular, renal. And in the second year you revisit each theme but with a pathological perspective. So you do normal physiology with each, and then you revisit it with pathology. And usually the people who are instructors are teaching very specific knowledge about an organ system so they're usually specialists. (Lance, second-year medical student)

. . .

Your training leaves you with the impression that care is very fragmented. We have evidence-based medicine and health-in-society courses, but those are really broad. We have no comprehensive "medicine" course that brings it all together in a meaningful way. We have a clinical skills course that is the actual practice of medicine and that teaches you to take histories and blood pressure and things like that, and it probably helps a bit to unify things. But for the most part it's fragmented, and maybe that leaves a negative sense in people's mind about what primary care is all about. (Molly, second-year medical student)

The growing complexity of medical science and presence of sophisticated health care technology to use in practicing medicine pressure medical schools to turn their focus away from a more general, integrated approach to teaching. Instead, the emphasis is on creating an efficient pedagogic model that allows proper preparation within a short time frame for the specialized residencies that the vast majority of students will enter.

If you look at a medical school pathology textbook today, it's 4,000 pages thick. And if I look at my uncle's same textbook, put together by the same authors however many years ago, it's much, much thinner. And still, it's the same four years of medical school. There's a lot to know, so much is thrown at you in a fragmented way. You're taught pathology by pathologists, clinical medicine by a bunch of different people, you might have an immunologist teaching you clinical skills. (Daniel, third-year medical student)

The third and fourth years of medical school may be no kinder to primary care. During this time, when students are rotating through various clerkships to gain experience in a variety of specialties including primary care, the doctors with whom they come into contact play meaningful roles in which careers some consider further.

I had gone into medical school wanting to do family practice. When I did my family practice rotation I was less than enthused with what I saw. So then I thought of going into internal medicine, with the idea of possibly moving onto a fellowship. And then I did a pediatric rotation with someone who really inspired me to change my route and think of a combined medicine-pediatrics career. If you have a good mentor, it can make a huge impact on your career. Because this is a decision I ended up making in my third year [of medical school] sort of on the spur of the moment.

I've seen it here now with some of the medical students we get. They work with a great resident or attending, have a great experience, and then say, "This is for me." Having people who are enthusiastic about their work makes a great difference. It can turn people who might have been not quite decided about their future plans to a certain career. I mean, you're not going to change the mind of someone who's wanted to be a surgeon since the day they were born. But for a lot of undecided people, it can make a big difference, and can make people feel more inspired about going into a particular field, like primary care. (Rhonda, third-year medicine and pediatrics resident)

Sarah is a general internist several years out of residency who taught in an Ivy League–affiliated medicine residency program. She saw firsthand the way in which a primary care career is viewed by her faculty colleagues who teach on the different clinical rotations to which students are exposed in the third and fourth years of medical school.

So much of medical training is hospital based, and so many of people's positive role models end up being specialists. For people to go into primary care, they really have to make a gutsy decision. Because it's not something praised by your cardiology attending when you're in the critical care unit, let's say. It's like, "Oh, well you're going to stop your training? OK. That's OK I guess. Are you sure? You might be too good for primary care." And that's a hard decision, to stand up for yourself and say, "No, this is what I want to do. Good people need to do primary care." (Sarah, internist)

The setting also matters. Traditionally, rotations designed to give students experiences in family medicine, pediatrics, or internal medicine are situated in hospital-affiliated outpatient clinics that provide a less-than-attractive view of primary care work. These clinics may serve disproportionate numbers of uninsured, sicker, and noncompliant patients, and can socialize young medical students to believe that such a "high maintenance" version of primary care medicine is what their job would look like if they chose that career. Part of this is due to the reality that busy community primary care practices have less time to mentor medical students interested in primary care. In a volume-driven primary care environment, medical students can undermine the typical PCP's revenue-generating ability.

They [students] slow you down. I hate to say that, but it's true. I would love to have students with me all the time and I do take students on occasion. But they are a lot of work, and you have to interact with them a lot. Your day slows down, and you get backed up because of it. And when you're trying to keep your visits on schedule, in a certain time frame, a student can want to talk to the patient too much and won't know how to direct the interaction, so then you're in there [the exam room] for a long period of time. (Rose, internist)

. . .

I'd love to take on more students. I'd love to teach more. But financially it's not feasible. (Frank, internist)

Another aspect of medical training that undermined the appeal of primary care was in how residents in primary care fields like medicine and pediatrics got exposed to general primary care. While family practice residencies have to provide heavy doses of exposure to ambulatory care medicine, and are likely to place residents for long periods in clinics and offices where they get a chance to see the same patients over time, internal medicine and pediatric residency programs often give only partial exposure to general outpatient medicine. The reality of separation between primary care residency programs and the realities of a contemporary health system where most care has moved from the hospital to ambulatory setting has been noted.[17] For example, most medicine residency training is still done in the hospital, or in the hospital-affiliated clinics noted above. Medicine residents interviewed felt that they wanted to gain exposure to the work variety and care continuity often associated with primary care medicine, and that this was not easily done in their everyday training.

I don't feel we get a ton of exposure to primary care. Even being in a primary care setting one full day a week, I don't think that gives you a feel for it. To really know what it's like, to practice it full time. And that's one of the frustrations, to only be there a day a week. You don't get a chance to know how the system works. And you may have some patients you have continuity with, but a lot you won't have continuity with. And you don't have control over the setting at all, over how the practice is run and managed. (Gabrielle, third-year internal medicine resident)

. . .

I think my residency was trying to push primary care, because we have much more outpatient experience now than ten years ago, two half-days a week and a month each year, in an office-based setting. [My] residency experience consisted of two clinics in internal medicine, both at the hospital's primary care clinic. And the problem with the primary care clinic is that we had mostly walk-ins, as opposed to ongoing care with the same patients over time. You would see the colds. You would see the sore throats. You wouldn't really get a lot of your own patients that you would see routinely. So I could see how that would turn a lot of people off. Actually, as I think about it now, that may have been one of the main reasons most of my co-residents in internal medicine didn't want to do general primary care. Because all you're seeing are basic acute illnesses and complaints that become fairly routine. (Harry, internist)

Sarah, the young internist who had taught in a medicine residency program, echoed what anecdotally has been talked about in the literature about the problems with the existing structure of primary care training in internal medicine.

A huge problem is that a lot of residency education for primary care, especially internal medicine, is in the medical clinic, which is attached to the hospital, and there's not much opportunity to spend time in a suburban or private practice where you actually have patients who do what you ask them to, and say thank you, and get better. You get a lot fewer positive experiences. You have a lot of patients in the clinic that might be uninsured and are trying to do the right thing, but you can't get them any services or medications. You have patients that just come in and want to be fixed up quickly for whatever is wrong with them, but don't really have an interest in taking care of themselves in a way that would help prevent them from having these acute things they're coming in for. And then you get patients with big psychiatric or addiction problems. That's not a fun environment to work in.

And not enough time is devoted to the clinic anyway, so people don't really get continuous care experiences with patients. It's supposed to be a continuity clinic, and the residency accrediting body says that. But it's not really. Because when you're in the ICU, you don't go to clinic. When you're on nights, you don't go to clinic. And we added it up last year and calculated that our residents were going an average of twenty-seven half-days a year to the clinic. That's not adequate. And it's an uncomfortable environment because you're not there enough to get comfortable. It doesn't give you the rewards you're supposed to get, following patients over time, for example, because you don't get to follow patients over time.

The entire residency scheduling needs to be reworked in terms of where time is spent. Because traditionally scheduling is done in blocks, you know, you spend a block of time doing this and then you move on and spend a block of time doing that, it's hard to think of how something longitudinal, like caring for the same patient over time, fits into that.

I think the entire ambulatory experience needs to be changed to get people to want to do primary care and, more importantly, to learn how to do it right. For example, some of the stuff I'm doing now I never did in residency. I never had patients ask about their varicose veins. My clinic patients could never afford an elective treatment. So do I know whether laser treatment or vein stripping is better? No. So I find myself looking stuff up a lot. (Sarah, internist)

Brooke, a third-year medical student, supported this view in relation to the third- and fourth-year clerkship experiences.

Students become really accustomed to seeing patients in the hospital, because that's where we're spending all of our time. And that makes us unprepared for what outpatient care looks like, or for what private practice looks like. Hospital care is such a small percentage of what primary care looks like across the country. It can't possibly be a good representation of what it means to go into primary care. (Brooke, third-year medical student)

In every medical school class and primary care residency, many individuals' career choice is driven by income concerns and educational debt burdens. But it is also possible that a higher percentage might select primary care if in these formative years of their training, which are the critical moments of socialization for young, aspiring doctors, more appropriate exposure to primary care occurred. Louise, a third-year medical student, intends to become a family physician despite feeling like her training has not encouraged her to pursue primary care.

If you're interested in primary care, you feel left out. There's so much emphasis on surgery and other medical specialties. We have a class advisor that goes over our progress every year, reviews our classes, asks us how we are doing academically and she always asks, "What do intend to do moving forward?" And when you say primary care it's like, "OK, fine, we don't have to keep track of you anymore." Like we can do anything we want and no one needs to keep track of us. And so we don't have to be competitive or have an actual plan for the future. It's like getting tossed off. It's nice in that way, like we have less pressure. But it's also like we don't matter to the people in administration.

They don't encourage primary care here. The teachers will say that primary care is important, but then say that this thing they do in cardiology is so much cooler. And they tip their hat to primary care, but do very little to encourage us as students to move in that direction. And by not paying attention to those of us who want primary care, it just feels like they think they don't need to prepare us in any way.

Most students may have some idea of what they want to do in medicine, but I never get the feeling it's totally close-ended. That they have made their choice 100 percent. So, I feel that there is room there. If something is presented to them as really respectable and really worthwhile and would give them a bit of academic prestige, that they wouldn't knock it out of consideration. (Louise, third-year medical student)

Medical training's inability to sell primary care and show off primary care careers in a favorable manner is a product of several key constraints. These involve a crowded curriculum, student perceptions and debt burden, misaligned work experiences for students and residents, and lack of appropriate primary care role models. But these constraints are not fixed forever in time. Some can and should change. Their existence, however, does allow medical schools and residency programs to exhibit a benign neglect in acknowledging the full range of the problem, and what their institutional roles are in solving it. The history of medicine demonstrates that the medical profession can shape the career choices of its youthful members, as well as determine which medical specialties assume prominence in health care delivery.[18] Why it currently chooses not to wield its influence in the direction of primary care at the level of training and education remains the larger, vexing question.

Differences between Younger and Older Primary Care Physicians

Older PCPs described their younger cohorts in a straightforward way that was consistent with how the latter saw themselves and their careers. Older PCPs understood that the younger generation liked medicine as a job, that they valued lifestyle and did not want to pursue their careers 24/7, and that they were less interested in "traditional" things like owning a practice or remaining in the same practice setting for more than a few years. Maura works part time as the medical director for a large primary care practice in the area. She often finds herself negotiating with young PCPs who have a definite sense both of their worth and what they want in these regards.

I think the young docs are much less entrepreneurial in their approach to practice. You have fewer of them wanting to come out and set up their own business. They want to find a ready-made job, step into it, and have a relatively high income. And that's not unjustifiable, given that most of them owe so much in debt from medical school loans. But they have a predetermined sense of what their income level should be, they want set hours, they want a lifestyle. They're probably smarter than us from that perspective. But I think they're much less driven to do this out of a primary intellectual and emotional love for the work. It's a career choice. It's not a life choice for them. Some of them I would go so far as to say it's not even a career choice. It's a job choice.

We've been softly interviewing for our practice right now. And we talked to one guy who said, "Well, I need this much money," and I said OK we can negotiate around that. And then he said, "How much are you going to want me to be on call," and these are first-meeting questions, mind you. And the kicker was when he said, "And in addition to my vacation, which I want to be the same as everyone else's, I only want to work 11 months. You don't have to pay me for it but I don't want to work it because my family goes back to my wife's home country every year to visit."

That's a typical example of what you see coming out today. They want that elevated professional lifestyle, that economic lifestyle, and they want someone to guarantee it. Now when I was starting out, you came out of residency and linked up with someone. You were expected to work for a relatively smaller amount of money compared to people in the profession with more experience than you, pay your dues, and then buy into the business and have ownership of the practice. Now, it's much more of an employee model. And it's hard to meet all of the competing demands around this. Because as the older cohort ages out of practice, there may be less of a feeling of ownership with primary care, ownership of the practice and the patients in the practice. (Maura, fifties, pediatrician)

Maura's perception was echoed by almost all of the older PCPs interviewed.

Younger people going into primary care are hard to come by. They want a set salary which sometimes is more money than I make and, frankly, the work ethic is not the same. (Mark, fifties, internist)

. . .

Look, the younger docs, they don't want to work as hard. They're coming out of a training system now that sets limits on the number of hours they can work, they don't have to do hospital work or be on call all that often, and they want different things in their lives. They want to make money but not have to do the kinds of things I had to do when I was first practicing to make that money. Being a doctor to them is just a job. It's not their life. And something may get lost for the patient and medicine with that kind of attitude, I don't know. But it's much different than how we were raised to think of ourselves. The training programs have partially pushed this. Because now with the work-hour restrictions, you work a twelve-hour day as a resident and you're done. And that's how people are trained now. (Rick, fifties, internist)

None of what younger PCPs got out of their "decent jobs" was news to the older PCP group. But harder to gauge was how this view of younger PCPs made the group feel. Did they resent the value systems of the younger generation who worked alongside them? There was no evidence in the study that they did. Instead, there were feelings of disappointment expressed by older PCPs at how their younger counterparts thought about their careers. Some of the older PCPs had little faith in the ability of younger PCPs to provide the same loyalty, collegiality, and support as they felt older PCPs had been socialized to do.

Being in practice is being married. And among the original principles was that nobody runs out without taking a look around and making sure everyone else is not going to get hammered for the rest of the night, if there's an issue and someone gets sick, there's an issue in the family, whatever, you go and take care of it, don't worry, we'll take your call, we'll take your patients. I don't find the same thing among some of the younger people who have come out. Maybe it's because we picked the wrong ones [in our practice], the ones that never knew what they really wanted to do. Nobody wants to live the lifestyle that we lived when we got into this. We don't want to live it. But unfortunately sometimes we're forced to do that. (Mark, fifties, internist)

Older PCPs also felt that younger PCPs were less committed to establishing a long-term clinical practice in the same geographic location that would result in seeing the same patients over many years. The larger statistics support them in this regard, as younger physicians generally move around in jobs much more frequently in the early twenty-first century.[19] Indeed, many switch jobs at least once within the first few years of practice.[20] For many older PCPs, their own allegiance to a single practice setting and the same colleagues was a vital part of their career identity.

When you came out years ago, the goal was to work hard and build up a practice. Now, if somebody develops a practice over two years, gains established patients, then packs up and says, "I'm moving on," that's unsatisfying for everyone. But you see it a lot more now than you used to. Very detrimental to the specialty of primary care, to its image. In order to get the full satisfaction of being in primary care, you've got to build a practice and be willing to stick it out. (Francis, fifties, family physician)

Despite these misgivings, older PCPs empathized with their younger colleagues. They believed that the younger doctors had little choice but to embrace primary care as a good job with varied personal rewards but limited appeal as an all-consuming endeavor.

All of the complexities now in primary care, the insurance stuff, the numbers you have to maintain to make ends meet, there are a lot of negatives for someone coming into this field today. (Brad, sixties, internist)

. . .

If you want it to be a commodity, fine, let's make it a commodity. You want to make it like going to the supermarket, OK, well then I close too, just like the supermarket. So, if that's what young physicians only see, I don't blame them for thinking of themselves in that way. (Rick, fifties, internist)

Ironically, some in the older group spoke of their own adaptations to the primary care workplace of today in ways that sounded similar to the lifestyle-focused adaptations of young PCPs.

Look, there's balance in life too. I try and make a balance between having time and money and family. I could work five days a week instead of four and make 20 percent more than I do. But I choose not to, because I like having a day off to do things I like to do like biking or skiing. Spending time with the kids. A lot of physicians I know are going to reduced work schedules. Because it's a lot to work five days a week. Just the hours you put in each day, and the amount of time talking and listening to people, the stuff you have to do now when you're in the office, I'd burn out doing five days a week. (Greg, fifties, internist and pediatrician)

. . .

We try to finish up our patient schedules by five or five-thirty each day. Because it's important for all of us to go home and spend time with our families. (Steven, fifties, pediatrician)

Regardless of the different belief systems or views held by younger and older cohorts, older doctors generally are responding to today's changing medical workplace in ways not altogether different from their younger colleagues. This result calls into question whether young and old are much different when faced with similar circumstances in their everyday work lives. Like some younger PCPs, an increasing number of older physicians generally work part time for less pay.[21] Many of these older physicians are male, over sixty, and cite reasons such as new and different job duties, retirement planning, or activities not related to medicine as their motivations for part-time work.[22] Several older PCPs in the present study also worked reduced schedules for lower pay, expressing a desire for more free time outside of work.

As we saw, less than a couple of handfuls of PCPs interviewed, regardless of age, still took care of their patients in the hospital, though at an increasingly decreased rate. Call schedules across both the younger and older PCP groups were less frequent than those of a decade or more ago as described by the latter group. Both the younger and older cohorts did few procedures in their offices, regardless of how much prior experience they had accumulated in performing them. In short, the realities of a narrowing scope of work, larger physician groups that could disperse call responsibilities, and economic imperatives that forced all PCPs to maximize office-visit time made older PCPs adjust similarly to their younger counterparts.

The Iron Cage of Pragmatism for Younger and Older PCPs

By similarly adapting to changes in the surrounding work context, both groups came across as highly pragmatic in fitting themselves to primary care jobs as they look now. However, this pragmatism had consequences for each group that shaped their relationships with work and career. Older and younger PCPs were survivors in making the best of their jobs. As a group, older PCPs were more ambivalent and dissatisfied with their work and career than younger PCPs. In many instances, these feelings were expressed subtly, perhaps through a wistful add-on during an interview response or through nostalgic comparisons to the past.

> I'm making less money now, and working harder, than I did ten years ago. That just doesn't seem right, and I don't understand it. I think back to the days I worked in an HMO, when some of my colleagues thought I was nuts, and I think what a much happier time I had then. (Quentin, family physician)

Some older PCPs had a difficult time making sense of the changes wrought on their work. While it was easy enough to articulate the specific differences, such as why hospital medicine was sacrificed, it was difficult for them to understand who or what was to blame. Very often, the enemy was external stakeholders.

> The insurers have been squeezing and squeezing me for years. Cutting my reimbursements, paying me less for the same thing. Medicare is paying me less now for things I do. And I can't keep practicing in this kind of hostile environment, where primary care gets no consideration. (Rick, internist)

Their tendency to focus outward distracted the older group from seeing how they were active participants in the restructuring of their work and careers. True, their brand of pragmatism was driven by a series of Hobson's choices that forced specific changes to survive economically within a changing primary care business model. For example, give up hospital work that was intellectually stimulating but unprofitable or continue to do this work but see fewer patients in the office, where reimbursement is higher, and hurt the practice financially. Join larger practices and share revenue with more physicians, in addition to pledging allegiance to a corporate entity and giving up personal control, or maintain control but potentially be overwhelmed competitively by others in the marketplace. Invest in and learn how to use unfamiliar, expensive technology such as electronic medical records, or be perceived as behind the times and lose patient business and extra financial incentives from insurers in the future.

Yet, in a tangible way, older PCPs, many of whom had been in smaller, self-employed practices at one point in their careers, adapted practically and proactively to the pressures placed on their jobs, lessening the effects of what could turn into worse economic and clinical situations for themselves. Theirs was a rational response to a restructured work environment. Older PCPs cast many of the adaptations to their work as desperate choices, instead of voluntary ones to enhance compensation or survival chances. As they discussed these choices, older PCPs lamented what they felt was lost from adapting "successfully" in their practice and career. In their minds, the losses included less intimate knowledge of patients and their families, less connection with other physician colleagues in the hospital and larger community, less prestige from the public for their work, and less stimulating, varied work on a daily basis. For older PCPs, the volume-focused, office-based workday did allow them, like younger PCPs, to earn a decent salary, come and go at a decent hour, have less call and more free time, and create clear boundaries between work and personal life.

But working in a job that for years forced many older PCPs to place their careers ahead of lifestyle concerns led some to express dissonance about their new job-related benefits. For instance, there was a collective guilt expressed among the older sect, especially male PCPs, that primary care jobs were now seen by younger doctors as "lifestyle-friendly." In talking with older PCPs, I got the sense that they fell into several camps: those playing the game as best they could until they could retire, increasingly puzzled about their misfortune to have worked during a time of such profound change in primary care; those finding some positives in all the change, perhaps working less or rediscovering pursuits that fell outside of work and career; and those moving strategically to situate themselves and their work in a way that would allow them to succeed in the brave new world of primary care. With few exceptions, none came across as all that comfortable or accepting of the manner in which their work was now performed.

Younger PCPs as a group were more satisfied and comfortable with their jobs. In part, this was the result of having been in active practice for only a few years. Whether or not their prolonged exposure to the primary care jobs of today would lessen that satisfaction over time is something worth asking. From the standpoint of a small, cross-sectional study, there is no way of knowing the answer to this question. But it is plausible to assume that since this group was familiar only with the type of workday that has formed the basis for primary care since the late 1990s, one defined solely by office-based work, fifteen-minute patient visits, jam-packed schedules, and visit-only reimbursement, the lack of comparative experience to something different or past was the real blessing in this instance. There was no nostalgic tendency in the younger PCP group and no personal upheaval from learning new ways to enact their work and careers. It was because of this that they seemed better able than older PCPs to accept and even embrace the way primary care jobs now looked. The current world was the only one they knew.

The experiential difference between the two groups is also a reason why some older PCPs expressed mild resentment toward the younger cohort and a presumed value system they believed was less than their own. As discussed, there was good evidence that younger PCPs were motivated to embrace the current primary care reality because of a perceived better fit between it and their own career preferences and expectations. Their motivations for wanting a particular type of career enabled them to readily accept the way primary care jobs were now structured, even if there were negative aspects on which to ruminate. But if older PCPs made Hobson's choices, perhaps the younger group accepted Faustian bargains that provided them with immediate gratification for the lifestyle they wanted but over the longer term could further undermine their collective control and scope of work. For younger PCPs who were the future of primary care, the willingness to give up or not take back complex aspects of their work, like hospital medicine, combined with a personal desire for a work week that emphasized clear boundaries between work and nonwork life, lessened their future ability to assert their own importance within a health care system that was doing everything possible to undermine the utility of the generalist physician.

In the bigger picture, young PCPs express mindsets not unlike the younger doctors generally today and, perhaps, similar to many of us who entered the workplace after the baby boomer generation. The view of medicine or any job as an "all or nothing" calling does not hold anymore for a large percentage of the younger cohort. Medicine is a rewarding career and well-paying job for those lucky and smart enough to earn the right to practice it. It is still a highly prestigious occupation in our society. But it is not, nor may it ever be again, the kind of idealistic endeavor that provides a seductive combination of prestige, profit, and unfettered autonomy that would compel a person into devoting every waking hour to it.

> I do think there is something to be said for the work ethic that was there before in primary care. I see all these older docs out in the community, taking care of their businesses, still doing a lot of call, going to the hospital, and I say wow. It was kind of commonplace when these docs went into it, to expect to work eighty or ninety hours per week. That's just what was expected of you. And today, whether it's more because medicine has changed, like tons of paperwork and things hanging over your head like medical liability, it's also just not the same job it used to be. I don't know if that plays a role in how much the younger ones are willing to do, put into it. For me, I think it does affect how far I'm willing to go, especially when I consider all these other things I want out of my life. I wonder, and I'll use a baseball analogy, when you talk about the number of home runs people hit back then versus how many they hit now, well, it's not the same game, so you can't really compare it. (Paul, family physician)

The game has changed. It is perfectly reasonable to expect the players to change with it.

Chapter 7

Women in Primary Care

MomMD.com bills itself as "a professional and social networking site for women in medicine" and "the most active online community for women physicians, medical students and premedical students."[1] Launched in 1999, the site contains an exhaustive array of resources, clinical information, discussion blogs, articles, job postings, products, and other features designed to help female doctors and doctors-in-training navigate their daily lives. MomMD is geared to mothers in medicine. Lots of active blogs on MomMD deal with a range of topics from family and parenting to advice about becoming a doctor to being a female medical resident. The blogs contain tens of thousands of individual postings, meaning that a lot of women doctors had used the site to connect with the broader community of their peers. MomMD is a virtual meeting place that helps you share your trials and tribulations as a woman doctor, if only to commiserate. Consider a composite exchange compiled from several similar discussions listed on a MomMD blog:

> I've been married seven years, and I'm a twenty-nine-year-old second-year med student. I was thinking that trying to get pregnant in second year might be ideal. Then I would know I was pregnant when planning my third-year rotations, and I could have my baby sometime during my vacation month in the third year. Even better, the baby would be a few months old when the residency interviews started. I figured that waiting until residency or afterward to have a baby wouldn't be good since the work commitment gets bigger. Does anyone have an opinion on this? (Blogger 1)
>
> . . .

It could work. But how intense are your school's rotations? It varies a lot. My school is more relaxed about it, but others aren't. It's difficult to do twelve hours a day and call in your third trimester or with a brand new baby at home, if that's when you have to do it. And breastfeeding or pumping breast milk is tough when you're running from one end of the hospital to another. Some people think waiting until the easier fourth year is better, but then there's the problem of traveling to residency interviews as you pointed out. There's no good time so do it when you want to! (Blogger 2)

. . .

I thought that third year might be better than fourth. I would have more time to spend with the baby during that easier year, as opposed to just being pregnant, whereas during first year of residency I would have less time. This is difficult. (Blogger 1)

. . .

When you want to have a baby, there are a dozen pros and cons for each possible time point in your medical training, and the cons all seem not so great! I'm also in my second year, nearly thirty-one years old. My plan was similar because I knew that I could take time off in my program and follow that with a mandatory stint of doing clinical research during third year. However, that means that I'm either pregnant during the tough core rotations (which are eighty hours a week where I am) or trying to nurse and adjust to motherhood when I'm trying to do those weeks. You're right, it would be nice to not have to worry so much about residency interview traveling and have over a year to spend with baby before the residency starts. But if you wait until fourth year, your pregnancy and nursing are probably easier to manage. My issue now is leaving a kid for most of their waking hours during residency. I've seen what the intern year has done to colleagues who don't have kids, and it's tough to choose to put a child through that. But if I wait, then there are other issues, like I'll be getting old! (Blogger 3)

When Rose went to medical school, MomMD did not exist. In fact, there were few female colleagues with whom to share experiences, fears, and best-laid plans at lunchtime, over the phone, in the classroom, or on the hospital wards. At the time, discussing when to have a baby would have been less important to women physicians than effectively negotiating the structural and cultural barriers preventing full acceptance and equal pay within a male-dominated profession. Rose became a doctor in the mid-1970s, with only fifteen other women in her entire medical school class, and few out in local practice. Being a female physician then was at worst a solitary, Darwinian-type endeavor, and at best one that involved a small cadre of geographically close individuals circling their wagons to build viable practices and ply their trades. In either case, it was an environment dominated by men.

> It was very difficult. I remember having these two babies, and trying to be in private practice, and I remember one night just being very discouraged, overwhelmed. I was to the point of tears. I said to my husband, "I just can't do this, this is too much. Nobody has shown me how to do this." And he said to me, "You have to show people how to do this." It was very difficult. In training, in residency, there were a lot of barriers we had to break. We had a lot of sexual harassment when we were in medical school and interns and residents. And at that time, you just shut up. You didn't dare say a word, because your professor would just flunk you. There was nobody to go to and say, "This guy is sexually harassing me." I can remember especially surgeons harassing us when we were doing surgery, saying "Well, you're women, you wanted to be here, just put up with it." (Rose, internist)

MomMD reflects a larger cultural shift occurring in medicine, where women now are over one-quarter of the workforce and growing, up from less than 10 percent thirty years ago. It also is indicative of the increasing array of support outlets, peer networks, and career options available to women who are physicians. On the surface, much has changed since Rose's experiences of the 1970s. Women now make up the majority of medical school entrance classes, and they will be 40 percent of the entire medical profession by 2010. Women can become surgeons as well as primary care doctors. Women have opportunities for social networking unimaginable thirty years ago. They have children and adapt their careers to that reality, working part time and as salaried employees. Women physicians can feel like they are part of a movement, a dramatic shift within a prestigious, competitive profession, as opposed to feeling like exceptions to the rule.

Yet, as those interviewed for this study convey, being a female PCP remains no easy feat, especially if you want to have and raise children. Like other work careers, it is filled with gender-specific challenges, reproductively driven ironies, and lots of things the males who do similar work never have to think about. It requires choices not solely driven by work interests, but also by the current and future expectations of being a wife and mother. These challenges existed thirty years ago for female PCPs. They exist in similar form today for the young women in primary care. And they are magnified many times over because of the sheer volume of women now going into medicine.

Having more women in primary care presents a big upside for patients and the delivery of care. Women primary care doctors bring with them an emphasis on listening, and on the emotional and psychosocial aspects of illness that may on average exceed that of their male counterparts, which is why the female PCPs in this study felt that patients wanted them as their doctors.[2] In a primary care world where patients are sicker, have multiple chronic conditions, experience fragmented care through a myriad of individual specialists, and suffer from behavioral disorders in vast numbers, the best clinicians nurture, dialogue, and connect with patients on an emotional level. The research says that women primary care physicians are more likely to have the mix of personality and motivation to meet this demand.[3] Women are the future face of primary care. But the women interviewed for this study reveal challenges and paradoxes that must be dealt with in order to make that face a happy, satisfied one into the future.

Why Women Go into Primary Care

Medicine and primary care are in the midst of profound demographic change related to gender. In 1980, just over a quarter of medical school attendees were female. In 2004, that number was 50 percent.[4] Today, one quarter of all female doctors are less than thirty-five years old and only 17 percent are over the age of fifty-five. Presently, women go into primary care specialties at a much higher rate than their male counterparts, who gravitate toward specialties such as surgery. Of all current residents in the primary care fields of family medicine, pediatrics, and internal medicine during 2005, women represented 52, 70, and 42 percent of the fields, respectively.[5] This is in contrast to specialties like surgery and radiology, where women were approximately 27 percent of the total 2005 resident number in both fields.[6] In 2006, there were over 256,000 women physicians, and almost half of them were in a primary care specialty.[7]

Female physicians may be more likely to self-select into pediatrics, family medicine, or general internal medicine because these specialties contain work that allows greater personal expression for nurturing, communicative, and empathetic personalities. For example, a successful surgeon can have flawless technique but no bedside manner. A great radiologist might possess superior visual acuity but little desire to deal directly with patients. But to be a good primary care doctor in the manner described above, a physician must want to interact with patients in close quarters, talk with and listen extensively to them, and focus on their emotional and psychological states of mind. Women, the anecdote goes, are suited to medical jobs with a high interpersonal component.

> I think women go into primary care because there's some fundamental, nurturing quality that women have more than men do. I think it's more that there's something about their personalities, just like why you find more men in engineering. Some sort of genetic difference. (Sarah, internist)

> . . .

> I don't know exactly what it is. Women like to talk more, so that may be it. We also like to listen. We like to hear what's going on with other people. That's just a part of how we operate. (Susan, second-year family medicine resident)

> . . .

> For lack of a better word, I just think women are more "touchy-feely" than men are. Just because we're wired that way. And that comes through in medicine as well. And this is comparing me and my husband. He's also a really touchy-feely male physician. And I'm probably average on the female spectrum with it, because I don't hand-hold all my patients, for example. But there's still a big difference between us. And he'll ask me, "What are you doing in twenty minutes with the patients?" (Caitlyn, internist)

> . . .

> I tend to run behind most days. Because I don't like just rushing in and out of the room. I like to talk to the patient. I like to hear about what's going on with them. That's the interesting part of the job to me. To be able to hear about what a person is going through, what their life is like. That's where I get a lot of my job satisfaction from. (Camille, family physician)

Women also may go into primary care because other specialties such as surgery remain dominated by male-centric views of how people should train, what values they should possess, and the all-or-nothing career approach they should display once in practice. This belief was reflected in what some of the women in the study identified as the absence of female role models in nonprimary care specialties.

> There's not as much a likelihood that women are going to be mentored by other women in specialties like cardiology or surgery. And there are old men in some of these specialties that don't think women should even be in them in the first place. (Sarah, internist)

Although research shows that role models play a more important role in getting men to pursue primary care,[8] it was the *lack* of appropriate female role models in specialties such as surgery that women identified as discouraging them from pursuing these other lines of work, especially given the histories of ambivalence and discrimination toward women in these areas. In addition, many medical specialties are still practiced as daily endurance tests, performed in a manner where working longer and harder proves one's worth to fellow colleagues. For example, the norms of a practicing surgeon remain getting up and into the hospital at 5 or 6 A.M., performing surgeries several days a week for six to ten hours, and seeing patients in the office or on the wards until six or seven at night. There is room for little flexibility in such a schedule.

Surgical residents have even greater demands. Not only are they expected to be the first ones into the hospital each day to check up on patients, which may mean 4 or 5 A.M., they are expected to be the last ones to leave at night. They also must compete with each other for the attention of attending surgeons, and get into the operating room as often as possible, which often means being in the hospital at all days and times just to afford themselves the opportunity to assist on a surgery. When not working in the hospital, they are expected to learn something in whatever spare time they have by which they can dazzle superiors when the chance presents itself.

Specialties like surgery are opportunistic in that many students and residents find themselves gaining operating room experience simply because they are in the right place in the hospital at the right time. Women residents with young children have more limited opportunities to "hang around" if they also expect to be the primary caretaker of their families. Without good female role models, careers in surgery remained for most women in the study daunting, hostile career paths. Given these perceptions, and the reality of seeing as a medical student the everyday lives of those working in the surgical specialties, many women did not believe there was a way different from the accepted norm for taking on these careers.

Jenny is a second-year family medicine resident. She has seen firsthand how many women in specialties like surgery think and act, as well as the reality of what is expected of you when in these types of specialties.

Surgery is still predominantly male. You have to be real tough as a woman to go into it. I know that during my clerkship in surgery back in medical school, the female surgical residents and attendings, which were very few, were real tough women. They were brilliant, but from what I knew I would say 100 percent of them had a lot of issues, personal and relationship issues, trying to hold their family together. I did not feel the women who were successful in these kinds of specialties had the really rounded, complete life that I wanted. (Jenny, second-year family medicine resident)

The issue of lifestyle may be at the core of why women choose primary care in greater numbers. Research identifies lifestyle as a key factor determining why women medical students decide to go into primary care.[9] Lifestyle is important for all young doctors. However, there is much less understanding of why lifestyle is so important to women, and whether or not their definitions of the term differ from that of their male colleagues. These issues were explored in the present study. All of the female students and female physicians interviewed perceive that a general primary care career offers greater flexibility, time, and support for having children and caring for them than careers in surgery or OB/GYN. This view is consistent with statistics showing that female PCPs on average work fewer hours per week than male PCPs.[10]

One of the reasons I went into primary care was that it fit my lifestyle better at the time. I had two small boys. I felt it was going to give me some flexibility in my life, and some balance. I decided to work part time, and I had some different evolutions of my schedule until I could get things right. But even working part time was stressful. I had to round at the hospital every fourth or fifth week. (Jane, family physician)

. . .

I haven't decided whether or not to have children. Part of it is career. That's one of the reasons I wouldn't move away to somewhere else to train to be a subspecialist. My husband has a job here, his family here. He would move. But I would never want him to move. I've thought of going away and doing a fellowship, or what it would take to become a specialist. But if I suddenly decide to have children, it wouldn't work out. Being away from here three years. Even staying in this location, and doing primary care, I think about how difficult it will be to have children. But it would definitely be easier. (Gabrielle, third-year internal medicine resident)

. . .

My prior job at the hospital-based primary care clinic was great for having children. I got fully paid maternity leave, people were really understanding about it, and I didn't have to worry so much about moving my schedule around or missing some time if I needed to, because my patients could be seen by other physicians there. (Sarah, internist)

Women PCPs expressed a belief, anchored in their perceptions and observations from training that primary care work, with its implicit emphasis on the family, stood for values that aligned with how PCPs should think about their own lives and careers. In particular, they felt that primary care as a field was favorable to the joys of parenthood, time to raise children, and the secondary role of work compared to spousal and parental roles. In this way, the women interviewed believed that primary care consisted of a "family friendly" set of specialties.

> Knowing that family physicians value the family in general made me feel that if I went into this type of career I could have a family, and that would be respected. I could end up working part time and things like that. I think that's a big part of the reason I went this way. (Hannah, family physician)

Many young female doctors may desire a career that is family friendly. Although it is difficult to pinpoint exact statistics, two prior studies showed 14 and 38 percent of female residents in the specialties of OB/GYN and pediatrics, respectively, reporting at least one current or prior pregnancy.[11] Since the average age of graduating medical students is twenty-eight, residency and early career coincide with prime childbearing years for women. Many of the women in this study either had children during their early training and work career or were seriously planning for that reality. All of them felt, before choosing to do so, that primary care work was less hectic, open to arrangements such as part-time work and job sharing, and less likely to interfere too much with the nonwork demands of being a wife and mother.

Hannah is in her late thirties and graduated from a prestigious college in the Northeast that emphasized the kinds of premedical training needed to enter medical school. However, she did not become a doctor right away. She worked in a research lab for several years, got married, and had several children. As her children grew into toddlers, she decided to apply to medical school. She went to medical school while also raising her children. While she believed that she was interested in family medicine as a career from day one, she admitted that once in medical school she gave serious thought to becoming an OB/GYN, but did not in part because of the demands of being a mother.

The realities of an OB/GYN career which involved unpredictable work hours, readiness to treat one's patients on a 24/7 basis, and the need for doing surgeries at any and all times of the day convinced her that the lifestyle of general primary care fit better with raising two young children. Hannah now works full time, but has flexibility built into her schedule. She works as a salaried

employee, sees patients for thirty hours per week, works from 8 to 6 three days
a week and half-days the other two days a week. She also has a third small child
at home. Her husband has become a full-time stay-at-home dad, giving up his
job to help raise their three children while Hannah works.

Kris is a pediatrician in her mid-thirties with three young children and a
husband who works as a cardiologist.

> When I started peds, I wanted to go into peds-hematology/oncology. But
> then I got married and had a child during med school, and you know, it
> was a lifestyle factor. I went into pediatrics because I loved kids. But my
> first month or so as an intern in peds I just realized from watching the
> pediatric-hematology/oncology attendings working and their lifestyle,
> and their ultimate devotion to their careers, that this was something I
> wasn't really able to do, especially in the line of work my husband was in.
>
> So I chose general peds, stopped the idea of the fellowship, to have a
> better balance between family life and career. I've been part time since,
> I've never really worked full time. Which is due to family reasons and
> wanting to be a mom as much as a doc, and this was the best compro-
> mise I could find. Especially in a two-physician household, it's pretty
> hard to have two full-time physicians, and you both have career, career,
> career, and then what do you have at home? So I sacrificed some of my
> original career goals for the betterment of my kids and family. (Kris,
> pediatrician)

Carol is thirty-one years old, married, and has a fourteen-month-old son.
She graduated from a state university and immediately went to medical school
and then into residency. For the past five years, since graduating from residency,
she has worked as a salaried employee for a large physician practice. Like
Hannah, she also went into family medicine in part because she believed the
specialty would be receptive to her as a young mother. Carol works 70 percent
of full time at present, five days a week during the afternoons. This allows her to
spend time with her son in the mornings, cuts down on expensive day-care
costs, and yet still makes her feel that she has a viable family medicine practice.

> I set my schedule up this way just so I could see my son for a good chunk
> of time each day. Some women just take a day off, and work longer on
> their work days, but I just thought I'd never get home if that was the case.
> (Carol, family physician)

Other younger women in the study who did not have children anticipated
the fit of a primary care career with their desires to be an involved mother and

spend time with their families. Jenny's choice to go into family medicine was made when she got engaged as a fourth-year medical student to one of her classmates, although she had always known that specialties like surgery would not allow the balance she wanted in her everyday life.

Originally, my interest was more in OB/GYN. The driving factor for choosing family medicine instead was that I got engaged earlier than expected. I know that sounds weird. But that was the main reason I did not become an OB/GYN. I looked into the future, and saw that there would need to be a certain kind of lifestyle. I think if I hadn't gotten engaged, I would've gone ahead and done it. It suddenly just changed the way I thought and saw things. My near future now involved wanting to cultivate and nurture a marriage, and all of that. We don't have kids yet, and we're not planning on it soon. And some people might see that as giving up, as compromising too much. But I don't see it that way. I can't really explain it. But I think it's kind of a faux pas to be saying these things, like "the main reason I went into primary care is because I got engaged." People in this walk of life, people who want to have careers in medicine, we're driven people, we're type-A personalities. And you have to be ambitious and pursue these lofty goals. You can't do anything short of it, and if you do then you're not good enough, you're not ambitious enough. I didn't see it as a lack of ambition. It's just that when I got engaged my goals and ambition changed a little.

I grew up with a surgeon. So I was kind of automatically attracted to using my hands, doing surgical procedures and stuff. But I knew, based on growing up as the daughter of a surgeon, that I didn't want that life. For a bunch of reasons. For a woman, I think it has its own challenges. I didn't want that for my family. I never saw my dad that much when I was younger. Only when I was in high school, in my teens, was he more a daily part of our lives. As a student, going through my surgical rotations I loved it, I thought it was great. But I noticed that even with the new 80-hour workweek requirements, that specialties like OB and surgery really didn't enforce them. And they couldn't because it's just the nature of the specialty. I want to have a family, and with my vision of what kind of family and household I want to have, I just felt that it wasn't too much to give up, and that by doing family medicine I could still do a little OB and some smaller surgical procedures.

OB, even if you're not on call, you can be called in at any time. Surgeries are always unpredictable. I mean, you go into a procedure and it could be very straightforward or you could be in there for hours. And it wasn't a matter of dedication. But I just knew I never really saw one of my parents growing up. My mom really held both ends for a long time, and I was blessed with that. But I wanted to go away from that. (Jenny, second-year family medicine resident)

Female PCPs did not lament their career choice to go into primary care. To a person, they appeared at least moderately satisfied with their jobs, and talked about primary care with a passion for the things that were good about it.

It's always a constant challenge. If you want to think about every patient and what they should be doing, and what you need to be doing. (Rose, internist)

. . .

I like the strong bond between doctor and patient in primary care. Just knowing the patient over time. Trying to make a difference in their lives. I also like the intellectual challenge, and having those challenges constantly. (Gabrielle, third-year internal medicine resident)

. . .

I love the variety, getting to see new things and interacting with lots of different people. I like to do it all, and so primary care fit that for me. (Camille, family physician)

. . .

I'm someone who would be bored with specialty medicine, seeing the same things over and over. I like being able to see different things in primary care, and I like coordinating patient needs. Patients need someone they can rely upon in the system, and I want to be that person. (Donna, first-year family medicine resident)

Most of the women in the study could have likely competed as surgeons or superspecialists, had they wanted to do so. They were blunt and honest about the trade-offs involved in being a woman in medicine. They did not overtly claim to "want to have it all" but rather viewed their career choices as a pragmatic assessment of how they could meet multiple role expectations. For some, becoming a primary care doctor was an appropriate trade-off. And the decision to pursue a work career that ended up, at least temporarily, being part time or lower paying allowed them to fulfill their goals of having and raising children. Generally, women who work part time are overwhelmingly younger and do it because of "family responsibilities," as one large national survey recently found.[12]

Different Styles and In Demand

There is enough published research evidence to make a case that women physicians, especially in primary care, emphasize somewhat different things in their interactions with patients, compared to male physicians. One review of twenty-six previously published studies concluded that "female primary care physicians engage in more communication that can be considered patient centered and have longer visits than their male colleagues."[13] This communication involved "more active partnership behaviors, positive talk, psychosocial counseling, psychosocial question asking, and emotionally focused talk."[14] Other studies present similar findings, that primary care patients are more willing to speak to and open up with female PCPs and share more of their histories.[15]

Female PCPs have been shown to possess communication styles with patients that are less controlling than those of male physicians, focusing instead more on building positive relationships.[16] In short, women physicians, and women PCPs in particular, may do the parts of their jobs that involve communication, social bonding, and history taking with the patient in a consistently high-quality way. Because of this, the patients of female PCPs are more likely to reveal things about their lifestyles, care habits, and family situations which, in some cases, open the door to a deeper, more comprehensive diagnostic and treatment experience.[17]

Pragmatically, these particular differences may give female PCPs a greater advantage over their male counterparts for clinical situations in primary care that involve working with new patients, identifying psychological illnesses like depression, dealing with sensitive issues such as domestic violence and sexual abuse, and managing complex patients with multiple chronic diseases. Good primary care that emphasizes prevention and self-management relies on PCPs having full knowledge of patients and their situations. It also involves having a trusting rapport with patients where the latter believes they can open up to the physician. If, as research suggests, women PCPs are more likely to get needed information from patients, spend more time with them, and address the emotional aspect of care and research in greater depth,[18] then patient visits with women PCPs have great potential to yield insights that allow better care management over time.

The differences may also result, for whatever perceived reason on the part of the patient, in more satisfying office visits for primary care. Time spent with patients is a key predictor of customer satisfaction within the health care system.[19] In addition, the enhanced communication described above may place women in a more favorable light than their male counterparts in relation to the threat of malpractice, since the scope and substance of doctor-patient communication plays a meaningful role in how patients cope with, respond to, and recover from medical errors.[20] Knowing that female and male PCPs bring different strengths to bear on the primary care visit creates strategic opportunities for practices in matching the right doctors to particular patients.

Women PCPs in the study were aware of these differences and generally felt that the larger body of research was consistent with some of their own experiences. They believed that many male PCPs emphasized things like listening and the emotional side of patient interactions in their practice. They felt some female physicians were lacking in these favorable qualities. However, they agreed that for a variety of reasons, many patients seemed to prefer female doctors.

Female PCPs believed that one key difference between themselves and some of their male colleagues was that they tended to listen more closely and intently to patients, in the process spending greater time with them during visits, and emphasizing the patient perspective to a greater degree when in the exam room. The lengthier aspect of female PCP visits with patients has been noted in prior studies.[21] Part of what went into the ability to listen more was their belief that patients, both male and female, were also more willing to open up to them.

> I think the women docs will want to take more time with the patients, know the whole family, and ask about more things. And the majority of the male physicians here, these things are also their intent, but I think part of it is not a choice we have as women. We just do it naturally. I think more patients will open up more to a woman than a man. I've seen that all the way back since residency. In residency, with me, in a single patient interview, more things would hurt on a patient, I would touch things and they would be like "Oh, that hurts." They'd talk more, complain about more things. And the male doctor walks into the room and they're stoic, and they'll say, "It's not so bad." I think something in the psyche allows you to open up more to a woman. (Carol, family physician)

. . .

> People want women doctors. I can't tell you how much people call and want women doctors here in this practice. They want a woman urologist; they want a woman to do their colonoscopy. And I'm not just talking about female patients. Men too. I don't really know why. When I ask patients, they say "you listen more," "you take more time," but I don't know why. Maybe women are just perceived more as caretakers. Maybe a lot of patients are looking for their mother in a doctor. (Rose, internist)

A second element in this enhanced listening ability was that women PCPs said they liked hearing about other people's lives, as well as more readily sharing things about their own life experiences with patients. While male PCPs expressed satisfaction in their jobs with having continuous relationships with patients, female PCPs talked at length about a personal need to spend time with all their patients and know their family situations. They emphasized the social interaction part of the patient encounter in clarifying what made for a satisfying work experience. This was especially true where female patients were concerned. Almost all the female PCPs felt strongly that women patients especially preferred women doctors when it came to primary care services, and in particular when it involved diagnosing and treating both physical and behavioral issues unique to women in the everyday world.

> Most of my patients are women. We kind of went through the same life stages together, so a lot of us have the same life experiences. There's that empathy, that bonding, that willingness to listen. They'll bring up issues with their children, or something that's affecting their health as a mother, and I can relate that to my own situation. So I can give them things I've done to cope or address these more role-specific health issues. (Jane, family physician)

.   .   .

> Women like to talk to other women. We trust each other, there's a bond there. I'm their physician but then they also see me as another woman they can talk to. (Loretta, family physician)

Some female PCPs also identified a woman's general emphasis on the caretaker role as another factor that seeped into how they practiced medicine.

> Women tend to run the house, and we want everything in order. Give me a man who would think of what to get for groceries, or know what to do for dinner, or make sure all the laundry's done, and that man would be the kind of doctor who would definitely act more like a female in the role. I like to make sure everything is in order for my patients before I leave that room. Make sure I've addressed different aspects of their care, and not just their medical care, especially for the older patients. And we're like a wave in this way, more subtle. It's part of how we go about our daily activity. Whereas a lot of the male doctors will be more like boom, boom, boom, OK, I'm done, let me get out of here. (Susan, second-year family medicine resident)

For the women who went into private practice years earlier, when females were fewer and far between in medicine, patient preferences for female physicians were critical to growing their businesses.

> When I started in my practice, being a woman was a tremendous advantage. It was a huge patient draw, for both male and female patients. I was expecting women to gravitate towards me, because I do gynecologic care too. But I was surprised to find that many men preferred me because I was a female. I don't know if it's a little bit of homophobia, because some people have mentioned that to me. Or that we tend to be more nurturing, at least that's our façade. But a lot of men have said that they're a lot more comfortable with female physicians. Half of my patients are men now. (Theresa, family physician)

> . . .

> When I first went into private practice, and I joined another woman who had been in practice for a year or two, we became busy very quickly. It was amazing how people wanted to see us. Initially, it was mostly women. But very soon, it became their husbands, their sons, their brothers. It was not hard to get busy. It was very easy. And to this day, people call here, and we have four women and two men working, and they'll say they only want a female doctor. And we'll say, "Well, Joe Blow is available," and they'll say, "No, I want a woman physician." So once we got into private practice, the barriers seemed to melt fairly quickly. (Rose, internist)

Linda is a general internist in her midsixties. She owns a practice in a large urban setting and has been a solo practitioner for thirty years. Her practice has always been comprised of equal parts male and female patients. She believes that there is validity to the notion that, especially in primary care, patients typically form more intimate bonds with female PCPs, and that these bonds help guarantee a steady stream of business.

> The first day out in private practice my schedule was filled. So, yes, I do think there is a difference between male and female doctors, a difference that patients recognize. Sometimes it's hard to get men in to see a woman doctor, especially a woman primary care doctor. I've had women bring their husbands in kicking and screaming, and then the husbands end up turning around and referring all their friends and family members to me. I think a female primary care doctor offers some different things.
>
> For example, I take a very detailed sexual history on my patients. I really pry, if you want to put it that way, and once you go through something like a sexual history with a patient, people just get very comfortable

with bringing up anything that needs to be brought up. Most male PCPs don't take a detailed sexual history. Most male PCPs don't do routine gynecologic examinations in their offices. So the woman gets stuck having to have two doctors instead of one. I think women also listen much better than men. (Linda, internist)

Research supports the notion that females in general tend to downplay status differences between themselves and others,[22] which may also make female PCPs more desirable, especially for male patients.

With me, there's no macho competition going on. I think there is that barrier between a male patient and a male doctor. A lot of male patients won't want to admit to something because then it makes them look weaker than their male doctor. A woman PCP just takes the patient totally out of that situation. There is no competition going on between a female doctor and her patient. (Linda, internist)

Even some of the women PCPs who were salaried were aware of their value to the larger practice in which they worked:

We're a huge draw to the practice. I and the other women doctors, everyone knows a lot of patients come here because they know they can see a woman. So, that's why we're always in demand and never have a problem getting a job. It's just smart business. (Carol, family physician)

The Paradoxes of Being a Female PCP

The movement of female medical students into primary care does not guarantee that primary care is an ideal fit for what they require to assume multiple roles in their daily lives. Despite the perception that primary care offered several key lifestyle advantages over other medical specialties like surgery, how female PCPs pursued its "family friendly lifestyle" did place heightened expectations on them that were daunting and different from their male counterparts. By choosing a field of work that made it possible to gain some degree of scheduling flexibility, part-time hours, and reduced workloads, and by having many colleagues that accepted decisions to sacrifice, for example, work for child rearing, women PCPs inadvertently raised the collective expectation that they could pull it all off. This created unforeseen pressures on them.

That is one thing that's respected here. I mean, maternity leave is maternity leave. You're not a second-class citizen because of that. But then getting back into the flow of things is one of the things I had to have one of the other female doctors support me on, because the day I was back

I was on call for like the next week or something like that. And it was like, "Hello! She's not on maternity leave anymore but she still has an infant to deal with." For example, my goal was to breastfeed for as long as I could, but I just couldn't work it into my schedule. (Carol, family physician)

. . .

The bottom line is that you still have to see patients and the work still has to get done. For me, I try to limit how early I have to leave every day to go get my son. There is some understanding as long as it doesn't affect anyone too much in a negative way. There's a lot of "oh yes, I know you have Joseph, and you have this and that, and you're a young mom and so on and so forth, but still, can you cover me or see my patients because I have to do this, that, or the other thing." So, there is some understanding, but I don't know if it's really working together to accommodate people like me. And I try to limit certain things because then it looks like I'm not pulling my weight in the practice. (Wanda, pediatrician)

. . .

Having children is incredibly stressful. One of my coworkers at my last job did a survey of women residents of their ideas about various stuff. Reading the survey responses would just break your heart. The amount of stress. My generation is the first to grow up after our parents, who were part of women's liberation, and now we can do everything. So then you go through school and you do really well and you excel, and then the idea of leaving all that, your career, to get married and have children, is very, very stressful. (Sarah, internist)

As primary care physicians, they could make an honest attempt to have a viable work career, have and raise children, and be active spouses and mothers. But the amenability of a primary care career to these other social roles fostered an implicit pressure that the roles could be assumed in their fullest form and simultaneously. While the role of primary care doctor could be modified to be consistent with their choices, other roles such as wife and mother were less easily manipulated. Because in the eyes of female PCPs, these latter roles still conformed to a traditional view that saw the woman, regardless of whether or not she was a doctor, as the homemaker, caretaker, and matriarch.

I think it's pretty overwhelming today. I see our new partner, who just had a baby a few months ago, and has two at home. Sometimes I walk into her office and I see papers piled up on her desk. And she's trying to rush home to breastfeed the baby, pick up the child from day care. I just sense that constant tension, that feeling of being overwhelmed. And that's what I felt, too, back when I had young children. (Jane, family physician)

. . .

I know my husband would stay home if we had a child. He's said he's willing to do that, and could do that. But I wouldn't want that. I wouldn't be able to not put in the time to care for my child, and I wouldn't want him to do it for me. But it makes me hesitate to have a child. Because I see how hard it is for some women. I have a friend, another resident, who had to send her child back to Puerto Rico, to live with her parents there, because she couldn't do it. I don't want to have anything like that. (Gabrielle, third-year internal medicine resident)

Both Carol and Wanda felt the pressure of fulfilling the traditional roles of wife and mother. They were two highly successful women, having competed and succeeded in the most prestigious profession on earth, who were working hard, yet they still felt the pressure of taking charge of necessary home and family demands. Carol was married, with an infant, and had a husband who was supportive and available. Wanda was a divorced, now single mom, caring for her son, and working full time. Like other women in the study, Carol and Wanda faced identical struggles in their attempts to take advantage of the "lifestyle" offered them by a primary care work career.

One of the things is that the woman's role is to drive other things that have to happen in the household. And I feel that besides being the one who works and earns the most, I'm also the one that has to do the other things like the groceries, sending out all the bills, etc. And we try to break up these other roles, but it's always a constant source of frustration. It's a little bit weird for sure. Cooking is a big thing I've had to recognize is only going to happen as a hobby. My mom was a great cook. I'd love to be the one that made a nice dinner every single night, and we sat down and had it.

My mother-in-law, who is very traditional, straight from Italy—she could care less that I'm a doctor. That's not impressive to her because I don't cook him dinner. And the fact that I taught him how to iron his shirts and he does it, oh my god, that's like a big problem for her. It's something that's always a continuing goal for me, where even if we're having peanut butter and jelly we're going to sit down and have some sort of meal. Of course, it doesn't always work that way because the way I've set up my schedule it's become a lower priority.

I'm sure we'll try and make it more of a priority when my son's older. I know my husband would appreciate it, because his mom always made him wonderful dinners. I wish I could do it, but I have to recognize there's not enough time in the day. It's frustrating, because the work never seems to end. So I'm constantly working at home. I feel like I never get a break. If I'm not in the office or spending time with my son, then I'm staying up to all hours of the night to try and stay afloat. (Carol, family physician)

. . .

It's difficult to balance the home side with the work side. For me, being a single mom, my son gets out of school at a certain time and he needs to be picked up. I have to be out at a certain time, to pick him up. Then there's swimming and karate, everything, and in this area everyone is involved in stuff, and I want him to take advantage of that. And then there's just the time and involvement factor. As far as how involved you get, there's always something to finish up with work, notes or whatever. You can only take it so far. And it leads to staying up late. When I'm on call, which is all the time for pediatricians, sometimes there's no calls, sometimes there's four or five, my son gets sick of me being on the phone all the time.

Even on weekends, we just can't do all of the same stuff other families do. I lived with someone for several years. I worked full time and was the primary bread winner. You work long hours, and if you have to bring work home, like for example with the electronic medical record we have I can bring it home with me and update charts, stuff like that, when do you do that work? You get home, you walk in the door, and dinner is not made. You have to make dinner. And everyone's hovering around with this, that, or the other thing, hitting you with "here's what happened today . . ."

You have to spend some time and there's things like your kid's homework that you want to make sure is done, and then helping them with their homework if they need it and then getting them ready for bed and tucking them into bed and then getting everything ready for the next day. Putting all the dishes away, cleaning up the house a little bit. And you're at 11 or 11:30 at night starting to do your work. That doesn't leave much time for your partner.

For me, in my own personal home relationship it was hard to balance that. We had a lot of arguments about whether or not to get a maid. I know a lot of physicians who get maids. And, unfortunately the person I was with was less helpful with things like making sure there were groceries in the house, making sure dinner was made. I would come home late a lot of nights and there was nothing there, the kids were not fed. It goes into the gender role thing where the woman is expected to do all of those things. To be a full-time physician and work a full day, do all your notes, and get everything else done, it's frustrating. Because then something's got to give. (Wanda, pediatrician)

This view of lifestyle, with its juxtaposition of work and nonwork roles, was different from how male PCPs defined or sought to enact the lifestyle desire. As we saw in chapter 6, young male PCPs also identified primary care as a field offering a balanced lifestyle. However, their version of it was less concerned with how to assume other nonwork roles simultaneously through the course of a day, and instead focused on maintaining separation between a full work schedule, which satisfied income demands, and time for themselves and family at night.

Regardless of age or career stage, male PCPs did not mention having to worry about "getting the groceries," "making sure dinner was on the table," "cleaning up the house," or "becoming good cooks" in fulfilling their nonwork roles. Instead, they talked about "freedom" from having their work career be a 24/7 endeavor, and "keeping control" over their time. They spoke of freedom from excessive call responsibilities and hospital rounding, and how this freedom gave them time to see more patients in the office and also enjoy their families. They spoke of the ability to control the decision of when they could arrive at the office each day and when to leave.

To hear female PCPs describe it, work and nonwork obligations converged regularly. Female PCPs with children spoke of their average day in a harried manner compared to their male counterparts. They spoke of never having enough hours to "get things done" or to do more traditional domestic work such as cooking and cleaning, which many assumed were their roles to play. Male PCPs did not talk about or exhibit the need to have job flexibility or part-time work for child-rearing purposes or to perform errands, or to have accommodations near work such as day-care centers to drop off and pick up their children efficiently. There were one or two exceptions in this regard, but only one or two.

Many young male PCPs were also married and had younger children. Yet, the tensions evident in how female PCPs talked about lifestyle were absent in how the men described it.

I find myself taking work home sometimes, which I don't like to do, but I don't have enough time to finish it during the day. And so, I'll tend to do it while sitting in front of a ballgame on TV. (Sam, family physician)

. . .

I have a relatively easy lifestyle. But that's fine with me. It lets me do other things in my life. (Lou, internist and pediatrician)

Harry is thirty-two years old and working as a salaried employee for a large, multispecialty physician practice. He is married and has a three-month old son at home. Harry sees patients from 8 to 5 each day, but tries to leave the office by 5:30 each night. Whenever possible, he does not bring work home with him. Lifestyle was one of the reasons Harry became a primary care doctor rather than a subspecialist in his chosen field of internal medicine. He wanted a career but also a life. When Harry talked about going home at night and spending time with his wife and infant son, or about his workdays, rather than speaking stressfully about needs like having enough nonwork time to "get things done," or assuming duties such as homemaker or child caretaker, he spoke about achieving a separation between work and everything else in his life that kept him personally satisfied.

Two different lifestyle realities may be at play simultaneously in the primary care physician workforce of today. For male PCPs, it is first and foremost the ability to have unfettered time in the office to see patients and generate income, clear boundaries between work and nonwork time, and a life outside of the physician role that they can shape proactively. It is lifestyle through the prism of economic and personal autonomy. For female PCPs, especially single ones, these goals are also there for the taking initially, but as other social roles are assumed they become luxuries in terms of the ability to pursue them. With the assumption of spousal and parental roles, females' version of "lifestyle" ended the tidy demarcation between work and nonwork that male PCPs maintained.

Male PCPs spoke of time away from work as a necessary thing for their satisfaction, an active choice made in the pursuit of self-interest. Women PCPs spoke of it as a necessity borne out of their attempts to perform well in multiple roles, a knee-jerk reaction brought on by pressures that left them little choice but to attempt to fulfill a variety of expectations at once. They did not resent their lot. In fact, many young female PCPs with children were satisfied, in a cautious way, with the precarious balance they maintained across all their roles. For every woman in the study, with or without children, married or unmarried, having the time to be or become a mother, while also attending to the role of spouse and family caretaker, seemed important.

Female PCP Work Styles and the Primary Care Business Model

The differences in work approach and qualities exhibited by female PCPs come with a price. This price includes work that does not always fit neatly into the existing structure of everyday primary care practice. It produces less income for many female PCPs, who on average make less than their male counterparts,[23] longer than desired work hours not compensated nor compartmentalized from the time spent in engaging other nonwork roles, and a feeling that their work styles are not as valued by the practices that employ them. The paradox is that the things women PCPs emphasize in their work that are good for patients do not align well with the dominant business model within which primary care is practiced these days. That business model involves seeing as many different patients as possible in a given day, with higher numbers of patients producing greater income.

This paradox makes some female PCPs feel like "second-class citizens," as an interviewee labeled it, because within such a business model taking longer with a patient gets viewed by practice colleagues as inefficiency threatening the bottom line, not something producing higher-quality care. Research shows that women primary care physicians engage in longer office visits compared to male PCPs.[24] Several women interviewed, especially ones with less work experience, expressed self-consciousness in their workday when needing to spend more time with patients to listen to patients' family situations, explore psychosocial issues hinted at during the encounter, educate patients, and so forth. They talked about the need and desire to have longer scheduled appointments with patients. Others felt they got backed up more in a workday, compared to their male colleagues, because of their particular practice style.

Caitlyn is a thirty-six-year-old internist with two young children. She works four full days a week in a practice with five other PCPs. She knows that she takes longer than the average PCP to conduct a typical office visit. She believes that this is due to her desire to understand as much as possible about patients and why they are in her exam room, information which at times must be explored more deeply with specific patients. But her style of practice and the longer visits that result produces five to eight fewer patients seen and billed for in a given day compared to her colleagues, which affects the practice and impacts her financially.

> I don't think there's a value placed on a longer interaction with the patient because that kind of interaction requires time. And that time is on your own financial back. I do something unusual in this day and age. I see my patients in twenty-minute slots. And it's to my financial detriment to do so. I either do that or I run two hours behind, because the way I want to practice medicine is getting to know the patients, getting to know what they do for a living, what their hours are like, what is going on in their lives. Just getting to know the individual behind the illness. And from the comments I get from my patients, I know they value it. I'm not doing anything different than I always did when I saw patients in fifteen-minute slots. It's just now I don't fall so far behind in the day. (Caitlyn, internist)

Carol also gets frustrated because she runs behind most days. She sees established patients in typical fifteen-minute appointment slots, but finds that halfway through her schedule on a given day she is already behind. She feels her skills rival those of her colleagues, and that she falls behind because of more "high maintenance" patients drawn to her practice style. Her strong belief is that this benefits the patients because a doctor who remains in the room an extra few minutes, probing to see if there are other issues like depression present, produces higher-quality medicine. But she is clear that in her practice, which is experiencing financial problems, this more deliberate approach is neither understood well nor embraced.

> There's no recognition from the male physicians of the fact that because we're women, and a lot of people self-select to want to see us, and these people just by their nature and ours will want to open up more, that we will require more time. And there are a lot of male physicians that are very comprehensive and will also take more time, but even they can't see the difference. That just by nature of being a woman, it's more complicated to do what we do. There's no allowance for that. It's hard to make policies off of that too. Because then the guys who are working just as hard will say, "Well, just because you're a woman, you get extra time with people or something like that?" At least it could be a little more recognized. And maybe it's because a lot of us are part time, and we're getting full benefits, and so that's the allowance that we're getting, that we're allowed to be part time. (Carol, family physician)

Carol works Monday through Friday but only for several hours each day. Though part time, her workdays produce the realities of a full-time worker:

> I try to get everything done before I leave, but it's really impossible unless you want to shortchange the patients you're seeing, you know, and cut down their visit time from fifteen to ten minutes. So I usually have to bring home dictation, lab tests for review, and then look at charts. I go home, see my son for a while, get him fed and ready for bed, but then its usually back to work, sometimes until 11 or 12 at night. (Carol, family physician)

Jane's children are teenagers, but she remembers feeling the tensions evident in part-time work between wanting to do your job the way you saw fit, getting out on time, and still meeting role expectations at home, especially with small children.

The more patients you see, the more money you make, since things are productivity based. That's kind of the way it's been for a while now. But for every additional patient you see, that's more work in terms of testing, paperwork, etc. you have to do. Even if you're part time, you generate a lot of extra work for yourself. I always felt like I was doing 20 or 30 percent more than the percentage of time I was working and seeing patients. Always putting in extra hours, getting paperwork done, making calls. I knew when I was home, that I would have to be home 100 percent. (Jane, family physician)

The primary care lifestyle is considered "family friendly" but implementing that lifestyle for women carries with it two negative by-products. These are the intense normative pressures for female PCPs to engage equally and simultaneously in multiple work and social roles, which raises expectations about how to fulfill all the roles adequately; and the unexpected negative fallout from the unique practice styles exhibited by some female PCPs in the context of a business model focused on patient turnover. Lower pay, perceptions of not contributing equally to the practice's bottom line, greater job stress, and the intrusion of work demands on their nonwork roles, even as they seek to protect the latter, conspire to make female PCPs' initial expectations about a primary care career go somewhat less fulfilled.

The sense is that women physicians understood on one level about these negative by-products, and worked hard to minimize them. But realities like this are isolating for the worker. Many of the female PCPs had, in their views, supportive husbands who enabled them to navigate their worlds more easily than they could otherwise. Still, after each interview with a female PCP, I couldn't help but feel that being a woman doctor was in certain ways as constrained as it was thirty or forty years ago. True, many women are now becoming doctors and may soon dominate some fields in medicine, especially primary care. But, like the women in this study, each faces personal choices about what kind of doctor to become, how much to give to work and career, when to have children, and the types of wives and mothers they should be. Each of them faces subtler discrimination in a primary care workplace that is not economically structured to take full advantage of their talents, nor provide them full accommodation in accordance with their needs and interests.

MomMD is now there for commiseration and advice. But MomMD cannot give them tangible relief on a daily basis. Or make these difficult career decisions.

Chapter 8

International Medical Graduates in Primary Care

Brianna is a family medicine resident from India. Now in her mid-thirties, she followed her husband to the United States several years ago when he got a job as a computer programmer working for a multinational corporation. At first, Brianna worked as a research assistant in a lab, and then decided to pursue a career as a family physician. Brianna comes across as bright, energetic, and eager to have a clinical career. She has raised a young child, lived apart from her husband for significant amounts of time, studied and passed medical board exams, and actively sought out her current residency position to reconnect with the medical training she first received in her native country. She has a four-year-old daughter, for whom she cares while completing her residency. Her husband now works several hours away for another company and, because of visa restrictions, cannot at present readily move back with Brianna and his daughter.

This makes life for Brianna lonely and difficult to manage. Her daughter is in day care, and sometimes she takes her in to work. She has no family in the United States. At one time during her training in India, Brianna wanted to be a surgeon. But she felt it would be difficult to train and work as a female surgeon in India. She likes family medicine well enough, especially since it provides the opportunity to once again engage in patient care, which she values greatly.

Ann is a first-year family medicine resident who has lived in the United States for almost two decades. She was born and spent her early years in South America. She went to medical school in the Caribbean after practicing as a nurse for several years. Married with four young children, she has left her family in another part of the country to participate in her residency program.

Ann is ambitious and focused, like all the immigrant physicians in the study. She has a family but has never given up the desire to have a professional career. She sees her family infrequently.

> My children are not with me, they're with their dad. I'm going day by day. It's tough because I've only been home two times in the last few months. I hope to see them more, when they get breaks from school, when I have a little more time in my program. I've moved them twice, so I don't want to move them again. (Ann, first-year family medicine resident)

Jenny is a second-year family medicine resident. She was born in Asia but has lived in the United States since right after birth. She did not get admitted to a U.S. medical school on her first try, so decided instead to attend medical school in the Caribbean. She is now chief resident in her program. Originally, she was interested in OB/GYN but decided to pursue family medicine because of her desire for a favorable lifestyle. She also finds that family medicine offers her the chance to pursue continuity of care with patients. Although an international medical graduate (IMG), she believes her qualifications are equal to if not better than her colleagues who graduated from U.S. medical schools. However, she worries that the field of primary care suffers from a more negative perception when large numbers of IMGs populate its ranks because of the potential cultural differences between some IMGs and their patients.

Brianna, Ann, and Jenny provide needed services in their residency, which is housed in a hospital-based clinic that serves a largely inner-city, poor-patient clientele. A high percentage of clinic patients are uninsured, suffer from chronic diseases, and engage in high-risk behaviors that negatively impact their health. Many of these patients would not receive any regular care if not for the services of the residency program. These residents do everything from delivering babies to assisting on surgeries to taking care of all the chronic disease needs of the center's patients. Most of their family medicine resident colleagues in the center are also international medical graduates, and many of these are physicians born and raised outside of the United States. This is a fact of life for U.S. family medicine residency programs at present. These programs scramble each year to fill their slots with qualified applicants from U.S. medical schools. Increasingly, this means welcoming large numbers of international medical graduates (IMGs) like Brianna, Ann, and Jenny into their programs.

International medical graduates make up one-quarter of all practicing physicians in the United States.[1] They currently comprise 36 percent of internists, 28 percent of pediatricians, 18 percent of family physicians, and 25 percent of all current medical residents in the country.[2] IMGs are made up of two primary

groups: American citizens who have ventured abroad to gain their medical education, and citizens of other countries, like Brianna and Ann, who were born and
and now live outside the United States, or were born outside the United States
but are now permanent U.S. residents. Within the group of foreign-born IMGs are
individuals who do their residency training in the United States and then return
to their home country to practice medicine. The majority, however, remain to
live and work in the United States for an extended period of time after completing their residencies.

The U.S. medical profession maintains a mixed relationship with IMGs.[3]
During times of actual and perceived physician shortages, IMGs have been wel-
comed with open arms to both train and work in the United States. At other
times, both the profession and the federal government have sought to limit their
numbers to protect graduates of U.S. medical schools (USMGs).[4] The driving
motivation for such shifting policies often involves conclusions drawn from
the most recent set of physician workforce assessments. When these assessments say a physician shortage is imminent, IMG policy is more favorable, and
when they say there is a physician glut, the policy grows restrictive. That said,
the research literature supports the notion that IMGs provide an invaluable
service to our nation's health.[5] Regardless of whether or not they are practicing
primary care by choice, they plug the holes in our leaking primary care system
by becoming PCPs and then often practicing in high-need areas of the country.

Comparing International and U.S. Medical Graduates

The research literature on IMGs is preoccupied with whether or not they are as
"good" as U.S. medical school graduates in doing their jobs. Studies focus on
how IMGs compare with USMGs on standardized assessments such as medical
board exams and in the quality of care provided to patients. In general, the
studies present mixed findings. For example, those educated as physicians outside the United States have been found to score lower than U.S. medical school
graduates on the first two parts of medical board exams, which are taken while
in medical school.[6] However, the immigrant physician component of the IMG
group also has been found to score higher on these exams than the U.S.-born
IMG group.[7] The immigrant population may do less well on average on the
"clinical skills assessment" portion of these exams. These test a person's ability
to interact with the patient, take patient histories, and communicate around the
diagnosis. Some argue that the lower performance of immigrant physicians on
the clinical skills exam is less a reflection of a lower competence and more of
having English as a second language and being raised in a different culture.

One study of over half a million physicians practicing in the United States concluded that immigrant physicians have board certification rates as a group that are in most cases higher than U.S. citizens educated as physicians outside of the United States and, in several specialties such as internal medicine and emergency medicine, comparable to U.S. medical graduates.[8] Another comprehensive review of existing research finds no differences in quality of care provided by IMGs versus USMGs.[9] IMGs also appear to possess similar professional and ethical standards as USMGs.[10] Where differences in quality are identified between USMGs and IMGs, the research often raises the question noted above about whether the differences themselves are the result of differences in clinical ability or the fact that a large proportion of the IMG group consists of physicians raised and trained outside of the United States.[11]

Many of the IMGs interviewed talked about what medical school is like outside of the United States. In particular, they spoke of the hands-on, all-purpose training they received as medical students in poorer countries that suffer from shortages of doctors and a lack of technology-driven medicine. This speaks to another criticism offered in relation to immigrant physicians: the fact that by leaving their home country to do residencies and then work in the United States they contribute to a "brain drain" that further undermines their homeland's health care system.[12] This brain drain describes a process by which poor countries lose their most talented physicians who wish to train and work in other countries such as the United States. In any case, IMGs as a group believe that the early chance to get involved directly in patient care gives them a practical advantage over U.S. medical students, who fall low in the pecking order behind attending and resident physicians in terms of hands-on interactions with patients during their third- and fourth- year rotations.

> The medical boards were very hard; especially part one of the exam. Because when you graduate from a foreign medical school, the quality of the training is different. Clinically, you're way ahead, because you get to touch patients on day one. You get to practice on day one. It's much more hands on. Students in the U.S. don't really touch a lot of patients until they graduate and move onto residency. I teach students here in my practice and they often say when I ask them to do something, "Oh, you want me to do that?" And I say, "Yeah, that's how you learn."
>
> But on the flip side, the technology and fancy lab work, and all the machines, we didn't have that where I went to school. It was a poor country where I trained. But we got to see a lot of complex things that students here won't see. You won't see meningitis here. Where I went to

school in the Dominican Republic, it was a dime a dozen. You don't see tetanus here. I saw tetanus. You don't see diphtheria or measles here. I saw them there. It's different but we get exposure that gives us some level of advantage over U.S. students. (Don, family physician)

IMGs also feel that training in resource-poor environments, while not preparing them well to engage in the high utilization, high technology, pro-treatment world of U.S. medicine, gives them greater adaptability in their everyday practices.

I went to school in the West Indies. And the medical students there do so much work on the wards. Because nurses don't do things like blood work there. It's something they stopped once HIV came along. Essentially the medical students are phlebotomists. And sometimes we're orderlies too. We do a lot of the work. It's a good learning experience, to do all the things you end up asking others to do here, like put in Foleys.[13] Doctors don't necessarily do that up here, and neither do students. Patient care assistants and nurses may do that stuff more.

My clinical rotations were in government hospitals. Patients didn't have to pay for anything. But there was always a scarcity of supplies. I would schedule patients for hernia operations and it would be three years out. And a lot of time you would tell the patient to go see the surgeon and tell him you have these kinds of symptoms and maybe you would get it moved up. You just give them some symptoms that make it sound like they have blood in their stool or something like that. But that's the way it was.

I got used to as a student to doing the most I could for a patient with the least amount of resources. It was very hard to order an MRI or CT scan or any big test. So, when you run into patients here who have Medicaid or who don't have insurance, you think, "What can I do to make sure that if I order that test, I really need to order that test?" And where other people might be like, "I really need to order that test, I want to order that test," I might be a bit more patient and see first what I can do clinically. I might wait a month, and have the patient come back before I refer them out, to see if things get better. It's making sure to do the most with what you have, and not wasting resources. (Sol, first-year family medicine resident)

Many IMGs attend medical schools that are located in close proximity to poor, health-care deprived populations. The top five countries where IMGs working in the United States receive their training are India, the Philippines,

Mexico, Pakistan, and the Dominican Republic,[14] which all spend much less on health care than the United States while experiencing higher, concentrated rates of poverty. The lack of available resources, combined with competing priorities faced by many of the citizens of these countries, besides the need for health care services, makes physician training a challenge.

> I come from a third-world country, and there we are dealing more with acute illnesses. We don't have a lot of prevention that's well emphasized. People will go to a doctor when they're sick, not when they are well. Usually our primary care consists of viral illnesses, acute hypertension. I worked in a malaria-endemic area, and we might do some health education type stuff there. But there is no setup for prevention. All these screenings we do here. Lead screenings, cancer screenings. They're all good, but in my country people don't have the time to worry about getting all those things done. They barely can take care of themselves when they are sick. We also don't have insurance, everyone is paid in cash. You can walk in to see a doctor. But you have to wait in line. If you're lucky, you might see them on the same day. (Tammy, third-year family medicine resident)

As a result, IMGs coming into U.S. residency programs rely less on technology and more on their knowledge, experience, and judgment in diagnosing and treating patients.

> When I was in medical school in Latin America, basically you just did a history and physical and just treat with that. Here, you have the luxury of doing all different types of studies and CT scans, all of these things are very expensive and you don't do them a lot when you're in third-world countries. (Lincoln, third-year family medicine resident)
>
> . . .
>
> In my country, we have maybe five cities that have access to MRI machines. So, I had to rely a lot more on my own clinical judgment practicing medicine there. Especially being in the rural clinic, by myself. I was a resident practicing alone in that clinic, and I had no one to ask how to do things, or whether what I was doing was right, until I went home at night and could look things up. Now it's great to have all these machines around you, but I hope I would always rely on my clinical judgment more in doing the differential diagnosis. (Sally, second-year family medicine)
>
> . . .

I don't mind seeing patients that might be poorer, or sicker, or haven't been able to take care of themselves. Because I've seen worse practicing in my home country. People don't have insurance there either. They don't have money. They give you chickens or vegetables if you're out in the country. And unlike here, I had to go clinical in diagnosing people's problems. Because the patient had to pay out of pocket for tests and blood work, and a lot of them couldn't pay for anything. People on the farms had to raise money even to see a doctor. (Susan, second-year family medicine resident)

The question of whether or not there are advantages to having IMGs learn and apply their clinical skills in a way graduates of U.S. medical schools do not is an interesting one. Certainly, they have much less at their disposal to aid in their training. But does lack of exposure to resource-intensive, high-tech care mean that these individuals are not the equals of their U.S. counterparts? The U.S. perspective would state that using technology as a rapidly deployed substitute for correctly assessing patient symptoms and diagnoses produces both quality and efficiency returns. There is no doubt of the partial truth in this statement.

However, the overreliance by physicians on technology in their work is also one of the main reasons why the United States spends vastly more than any other country on health care, but still underperforms when it comes to producing a healthy population.[15] When speaking with IMGs about their resource-poor medical training environments I recalled that an older U.S.-trained PCP in the study had in an earlier interview addressed the differences he saw between a more "traditional" style of primary care medicine and the expensive, high-tech brand of medicine many PCPs in the United States now practiced.

The style of medicine being practiced today by a lot of docs, especially the younger ones, is much more reflexive—do the test, do this, do that. Maybe it's the time constraint. Maybe it's easier just to send things out. Either get a test done, or get a subspecialist involved. For instance, someone has a stomach pain, and they do stomach tests. How about listening to the story? I still do most of my diagnosing by listening. I believe you only do a test if you think it will change what you're going to do for the person. But I think a lot of the young docs now, someone comes in with a hurt shoulder and they're like, "OK, let's do an MRI."

And a lot of these things, like MRIs, you find things that aren't a big deal that you would've never found and had to worry about if you hadn't done the test. It bugs me because it brings on more and more tests. And people like the radiologists sit there and ring it up, chi-ching. I have one guy, with a pancreatic cyst, and the radiologist says, "Looks like a cyst, not exactly sure, repeat in three months." So the patient came in today, having had the scan repeated, and I said, "OK, here it is, looks great." And here is what the radiologist said, "The cyst is unchanged from three months ago. Would recommend one more follow-up in 3–6 months."

So everyone makes a little money from it. And the younger docs especially, because they don't have the time with patients, they figure this is more expeditious. And they may also have more of a rote thing, like, "OK, if this hurts you do this, if that hurts, you do that." They don't ask enough questions. They may jump to conclusions a little more quickly because of the time pressure. And they deal with the fallout later when the tests come back. (Frank, internist)

The compulsion to use any and all available means for practicing "quality" medicine was evident in how some of the IMGs now practicing in the United States talked about their current jobs. For example, Lincoln's perspective seemed to be no different from the USMGs interviewed, in that now working as a resident within the U.S. health system he believed that there were more advantages than drawbacks to having technology available.

Do I mind having the opportunity now to have all the things at my disposal? No, I don't mind at all. I mean, you don't want to go crazy with ordering this test or that test, but it's nice to be able to confirm more quickly whether you are right about something. In my home country where I trained, you got a lot of skill having nothing but your own analysis and judgment to rely on, and the patient's history and physical, but of course you never knew sometimes whether you were making the wrong decision.

And now, especially here in this country, with all the legal implications of making a mistake or not doing as much as possible for the patient, you need that technology to help cover yourself. Again, the patients in my country don't expect the same things the patients here do. The ones in my country are poor, they look at the doctor with respect, and they are happy just to get some kind of care for themselves. The patients here have much greater expectations for how you should care for them. (Lincoln, third-year family medicine resident)

For Lincoln and thousands of IMGs like him, it is an open question whether or not the added judgment and cognitive skills gained from working primarily with one's experience and ability to reason suffers once those skills compete against the use of technology and sophisticated laboratory testing as decision-making aids. As Lincoln points out, the U.S. standard of care necessitates that appropriate means be used in the diagnostic and treatment processes that physicians employ. The risk of malpractice is too great not to comply. However, for aspiring physicians learning how to do their jobs, a commitment to less technology-dependent approaches may produce future doctors who save the system money and reduce unnecessary burdens on patients. This is especially true for primary care.

The Pros and Cons of IMGs in Primary Care

Given the equivocal nature of the research examining IMG quality and competence, the bigger issue is the extent to which IMGs contribute to the vitality of the U.S. primary care system. Judging from the significant numbers of IMGs that now comprise the field of primary care, there is little doubt that this group fills needed workforce gaps in the delivery of primary care services, especially in poorer urban and rural areas of the country. Less than 50 percent of USMGs now choose a primary care specialty for their residency training, and this figure includes the high percentage of residents who will end up subspecializing within medicine and pediatrics, rather than become generalists. This is down from almost 75 percent twelve years ago. IMGs comprise over one-third of both family practice and internal medicine residents, and a quarter of pediatric residents.[16] In particular, the percentage of IMGs in family practice residencies has increased substantially over the past decade, mainly because the specialty is not perceived as attractive to significant numbers of USMGs.[17] The 2007 National Resident Match saw 38 percent of the 2,313 positions in family medicine filled by IMGs, with 23 percent of the IMG group comprised of immigrant or foreign-born IMG physicians.[18] In the past decade, the number of U.S. medical students choosing family medicine as a specialty has declined over 50 percent.

IMGs are perhaps the most important group of safety net providers in the United States.[19] They are more likely to practice medicine in rural and underserved areas of the country.[20] They also treat higher percentages of the American poor.[21] IMGs from particular racial and ethnic backgrounds may be more likely to practice within communities that contain significant percentages of their own ethnic groups.[22] They staff residency programs in rural and inner-city areas in disproportionate numbers. Many end up practicing primary care for several years in these underserved areas.

The reasons why IMGs, particularly immigrant physicians, end up practicing both primary care and in underserved areas is twofold: primary care residencies are more easily obtainable for them compared to specialty residencies in areas such as surgery; and the most common visa obtained by immigrant physicians to live and work in the United States is the J-1 visa. The J-1 offers the potential for obtaining a waiver from the federal government that allows doctors to avoid returning to their home country for at least two years in return for practicing medicine in an underserved area in the United States.

> I really don't have a choice. I need to practice in an underserved area because I need my papers. I need my visa to be converted to a green card. (Sally, second-year family medicine resident)

For IMGs who are citizens or permanent residents, the need to gain entry into the United States is not the issue. Rather, finances and a personal desire to become a physician, regardless of where they receive their initial training, factor in their decision to work in underserved communities. Don is a practicing family physician, an American citizen of Hispanic descent who went to medical school in Latin America. He always wanted to be a primary care physician. He loves the variety in the work, the feeling that he is making an important difference for many patients who need basic services by keeping them healthy and capable of working. He values the long-term relationships he develops with his patients. But he makes no apologies for why most IMGs gravitate into primary care.

> For us as foreign medical graduates, we just want to get in. We'll take anything, we'll try and get in to medicine anywhere we can. And there's more residency slots open in undervalued specialties like family medicine than there is in specialties like otolaryngology. That's the big reason there's so many foreign grads in primary care. It's where we can get in. (Don, family physician)

Lincoln also feels strongly that IMGs are committed individuals but limited in what they can do in the U.S. health care system.

> Not a lot of the U.S. grads want to do peds or OB or family practice. If you ask them, they want to be cardiologists or endocrinologists or surgeons. Because these jobs pay a lot. As foreign medical grads, we have a lack of options, so we go into primary care. It will take a long shot for us as foreign medical grads to get into a superspecialty residency like cardiology. It can happen. I'm not saying it can't happen. But it's going to take a long shot. (Lincoln, third-year family medicine resident)

Both Don and Lincoln's first language is Spanish, and as a result both attract large patient populations in their practices that consist of Spanish-speaking citizens, immigrants, and migrant workers laboring for local farms and businesses. Despite practicing in a suburban setting, Don says these types of patients seek him out simply because there are so few Spanish-speaking family physicians in the area. Providing culturally appropriate care is one advantage many immigrant physicians bring to their work, and in a country as diverse as the United States, their ability to understand and connect with individuals of their own background increases the prospects for greater quality of care.[23] Immigrants now make up approximately 13 percent of the total U.S. population, and Latinos and Asians represent the two fastest-growing groups of immigrants.

Having a diverse pool of IMGs from which to draw upon in treating diverse patient populations is a competitive advantage offered by the field of primary care. However, placing IMGs who are immigrant physicians in clinical care situations where there might be language and cultural barriers with patients can shape the perceived quality of care provided in negative ways.[24] It also may decrease the level of job satisfaction felt by immigrant physicians. Jenny, an Asian American who went to school in the Caribbean, works with a lot of immigrant physicians. She has seen firsthand the problems encountered by immigrant physicians who care for patient populations that are different in terms of racial or ethnic heritage. At the least, communication difficulties, misunderstandings, and a more tenuous physician-patient relationship often result.

> I think it's unfair for the immigrant doctors. They really do face a lot of challenges as family doctors that have to cater to populations that are different from them. They've been on the receiving end of a lot of negative comments. I see that problem growing because of the increased number of IMGs going into primary care. And it's tough enough if you're a woman, and then maybe you're younger as well. And I've witnessed discussions initiated by some of my colleagues that because of language or cultural barriers, it doesn't come across right. And I imagine myself as a patient thinking, "What are you saying? I don't understand you." (Jenny, second-year family medicine resident)

While there is no conclusive proof that IMGs provide lower quality of care to patients than graduates of U.S. medical schools, patients may form perceptions that their care is substandard as a result of not being able to understand the physician.[25] They feel put upon to define or explain what they believe are things the physician should already know with respect to societal norms or cultural idiosyncrasies. Some patients are simply uncomfortable interacting with someone not sharing their racial or cultural background.[26] Patients expect their physicians to be experts. If patients feel they must explain or clarify too much, their overall level of confidence may wane even if the quality of the care provided is good.

For many IMGs, this tension between perception and reality is an everyday fact of life. The immigrant physicians in this study had strong opinions on how their unique racial and ethnic backgrounds might affect patient care. No one interviewed felt they delivered worse care because they were not culturally compatible or fully communicative with patients. Many felt they provided better quality of care for their uninsured and underinsured patients because they identified with their socioeconomic status, the type of challenges and existence they had, and because the early brand of medicine they practiced as students involved having to do more with less, which for uninsured patients without the resources to pay for their health care was to their advantage. However, they also believed that there were real cultural and language barriers that led some patients to form erroneous conclusions about their skills as clinicians.

> As a foreign medical graduate, it's hard for me to be thinking of a word in English, when I'm thinking about it in my first language. I can't really talk as fast as I can think. You're not born here. Sometimes it's hard to explain yourself to patients, and they get frustrated. Some patients are receptive, some are skeptical. But with the patient population we have here, I haven't encountered any racist patients that don't want to see me. Because the patients here are used to seeing doctors from a lot of different backgrounds. It's like the United Colors of Benetton. I have more problems with patients who think I'm too young to be a doctor, and they try and manipulate me more on that end. But if I can't put a word onto something I'm thinking, sometimes a patient might interpret that as a lack of knowledge on my part.
>
> But my experience may be because I'm in a bigger city. I had a friend who practiced upstate where there were a lot of white people. And they were more likely to look over their shoulder and say, "Who is this Asian guy coming in here, there are no other doctors here except him?" And he went into the grocery store with his secretary and everyone was looking at him. She said, "Doctor, you forgot to remove your stethoscope, that's why they're looking at you." And he said, "Do you really think they're looking at me because of my stethoscope? It's because of my color, and my face." (Sally, second-year family medicine resident)

Immigrant physicians admitted that language difficulties in particular posed extra challenges when seeing patients. Many immigrant physicians have learned English as a second language, but they may maintain heavy native accents through which that English is communicated. They expressed empathy toward patients who sometimes did not immediately understand them.

> My patients might tell me politely sometimes, "I don't understand you 100 percent, but I can figure it out." And I don't mind if they don't understand me, I just tell them to ask me to repeat what I've said. I don't mind saying that right up front, and I don't mind repeating myself. There are always patients that give you attitude, especially when you're admitting them from the ER, and they have psych issues. (Tammy, third-year family medicine resident)

Brianna, the family medicine resident from India, is very sensitive to how patients perceive her and other immigrant physicians because of their accents. However, even more important in her mind are the sociocultural gaps that exist.

> Every day I face these issues. When I was new, some of the patients could be mean. They would say things like, "You should probably go back to where you come from," and "what kind of English are you speaking?" And I would say that I'm speaking English, it's British English maybe but it's still English. And I don't have that much of an accent. And most of what I speak is American English now. But some of them made me cry. I don't understand if they're joking or not sometimes with me.
>
> Where I come from, especially for women, drinking, smoking and drugs are a taboo. We don't even understand some of the things they are talking about here. So when I'm taking the social history of a patient, a lot of times I don't understand what they are saying, so I have to ask them to explain it. And they think I'm crazy or something. Like I don't know what a joint is, and they'll say, "You don't know what a joint is? It's a joint." And my junior residents will laugh at me and say, "You don't know this?"
>
> So, I always have that problem and I feel embarrassed. And sometimes I don't know when patients are being sarcastic or some patients are saying some American jokes or sayings, and I'm like, "OK," but they'll know I don't get it. I'm still learning all those things, and I find them difficult. And some patients don't understand me when I'm talking, not all of them but some of them. So I have to say things again. People here are so sophisticated. When I'm trying to say something to them I'm not trying to be rude, but it sounds rude to them. A lot of us foreign grads are not used to it. You have to say "please" and "thank you" in every sentence and some of us are just not used to that. If you don't say "please"

they say you're rude. And I'm not being rude. I'm just not used to it. And sometimes patients react in a different way. I've seen other foreign grads go through the same problem.

At least my English is not bad, some other foreign grads, their English is bad. They also speak their English in the same tone as their language, and what happens is that they end up talking loud or in a certain tone and patients get upset. We had one patient, and one of the other foreign grads was going to go in and see them, and was talking in a loud tone outside the exam room, and the patient said, "I don't want to see that doctor." They completely said, "No, they can't come in this room."

And the doctor didn't mean anything by the tone he was using. I know him personally and he's a great guy. He just doesn't know how to talk. He knows what to say, just not how to say it. They think that this person doesn't have good bedside manners. But it's not like that. I don't want to be rude or mean to patients but it just sounds like that to them. I'm trying to get better at all this, but it's been a struggle since day one. It's funny, I never feel any problems like this when I'm outside my job. But in my job I do. (Brianna, third-year family medicine resident)

The cultural divide between some IMGs and their patients is a real issue. Can it be expected that physicians who have spent most of their lives in other countries understand immediately all of the cultural nuances of life in America? Many white, middle-class graduates of U.S. medical schools face similar divides practicing in urban areas with high concentrations of nonwhite populations. Do the same perceptions of decreased care quality pertain to them as well? It may remain more a matter of properly exposing immigrant physicians to the peculiarities of American medicine and different cultures early on, before they begin their residencies in the United States.[27] However, this would require the medical profession and medical education establishment to acknowledge IMGs as a major workforce group, especially in primary care, and engage them earlier in their training as viable providers of primary care services in the United States.

A key criticism levied against IMGs is that they are not truly committed to serving in a primary care career, but only interested in gaining a foothold in U.S. medicine so they can remain in the country and pursue nonprimary care specialties. This remains a cynical view. Many immigrant physicians are already permanent U.S. residents or citizens. And lack of interest in a primary care career defines the current perspective of almost all U.S. medical students. There was begrudging acceptance by some PCPs of the role of IMGs in avoiding a more severe workforce shortage. But there was less acknowledgment that this group plays a major part in solving the primary care crisis in the United States.

> I see very little interest in the foreign medical graduates, particularly the ones from other countries, in helping improve primary care. The cultures are different, and a lot of these foreign grads just use primary care to get into the system. Forty percent of the Match in family medicine the past couple years were foreign grads. And that to me is just like not filling the Match. You know, over two-thirds of people in this country receive their primary care in places where foreign grads don't want to practice. They don't want to go to some rural town in Iowa to practice, for the obvious cultural reasons, and I don't blame them. A lot of them take these residencies because they can get into them and then they go into something else. They would take a residency in podiatry if that was a way to get into the system. And so they don't really have an interest in anything being done to try and get primary care improved. I mean, they're very, very good doctors, but a lot of them go home when they're done, they go after other residencies, and if they don't they have a tendency to find niche areas like community health centers. They have no intention of becoming full scope primary care providers. (Trevor, family physician)

IMGs in the study did not apologize for taking advantage of the opportunity to gain access to the U.S. medical profession through primary care residencies and careers. Some IMGs in the study were interested in remaining generalist physicians, and others thought they might continue their training at some point in another specialty area. However, they realized how difficult it would be for them to do this because of the competition for these other specialties and the stigma associated with being a foreign medical graduate.

> U.S. medical students get guided every step of the way. They just have to pass their step 1 and they can go start their residency in a teaching hospital. Foreign medical grads have to rely on themselves. No one is there to help them. And I think this makes me stronger. I think I worked harder and I think U.S. medical grads have more advantages than me. I don't think I'm a better doctor than them, just that I've had to work harder. And most U.S. medical students don't want primary care. They think it's too easy for them. They all want to do fellowships, continue their training. I'm not worried about doing a fellowship. I want to practice medicine. (Sol, first-year family medicine resident)

The reality of what IMGs do for the U.S. primary care system should negate criticisms levied against this strategically important work group. Were it not for IMGs, the fate of U.S. primary care would have been sealed a decade ago. They prop up at least one primary care specialty's existence—family medicine. And it seems to be of little importance whether or not, if given the choice, they would choose primary care in significant numbers. Right now and for the fore-seeable future, they represent a significant portion of the doctors doing gener-alist medicine. There is little evidence they provide lower quality of care than USMGs. They are a richly diverse group culturally. They have received their medical school training in hardscrabble contexts that prepare them to care for poorer segments of U.S. society.

In short, they should be looked upon as a group that can help revitalize the field of primary care.

Part III

Fixing Primary Care

Chapter 9

The Medical Home

Primary Care Savior?

The most important idea currently touted as a model for revitalizing primary care is the medical home.

> The medical home label is like apple pie and motherhood. You can't argue with it. (Skip, PCP and health plan manager)

This idea is not new. First coined by the American Academy of Pediatrics in the late 1960s, it has been expanded upon, repackaged, and embraced tentatively by all three primary care specialties, large employers, some insurers, and by state and federal governments. In March 2007, the American Academy of Family Physicians, American Academy of Pediatrics, American College of Physicians, and American Osteopathic Association released the "Joint Principles of the Patient-Centered Medical Home." This document provides insight into the various elements of the medical home. The most important element is the pairing of each patient with a single PCP. Other elements include a physician-directed medical practice that involves teams comprised of all office staff with important roles to play; a "whole person" emphasis on care coordination and high quality; enhanced patient access to care through virtual communication enhancements; improved tracking and accountability for care delivered; and appropriate payment to recognize the added value of medical home type care.[1]

What this means in everyday practice for the individual patient still looms as a mystery. In theory, it would work something like this. Patients would have a single PCP to help navigate their care within any part of the health delivery system. This PCP would maintain detailed information on all his or her patients within an electronic database used for identifying individuals and groups requiring care. For example, such a database could provide prompt reminders to both physicians and their diabetic patients for when preventive checkups and blood work are needed. This database would be a repository for test results, clinical notes, and information from visits patients make to other specialists. The information in the database would be regularly maintained and updated, and the PCP could merge patient information across the entire practice to assess whether or not overall care is effective.

In addition, the PCP and practice would allow patients to access information and care in a manner most convenient for them: through the use of e-mail communication, Web-based education, and phone contact with not only the physician but other team members in the practice such as the nurse. Emphasis would be placed on helping individuals increase their ability to self-identify and manage problems. The care given to every patient would be based on sound, scientific evidence where available. Office staff would share the common goal of providing a satisfactory care experience, from the point of the patient walking into the practice to checking out after an exam-room visit. Both the PCP and the practice would be held accountable for making sure the total care experience was high quality. PCPs would develop and share comprehensive care plans with patients, and these plans would be monitored over time to ensure appropriateness. Patient perceptions of satisfaction with the PCP and practice would be very important, and the practice would be expected to report regularly to external stakeholders on how well they meet the right standards for their patients.

This is the vision of the comprehensive medical home. It is not a recycled form of the generalist model of primary care circa 1970 because it makes PCPs more accountable for the care they provide, gives patients greater involvement in their care, and casts the PCP as one important component of an overall practice team. Yet, in the broader strokes of forging a tighter, long-term relational rather than transactional bond between physician and patient, and making the patient an individual with unique needs instead of simply another "customer," the medical home and generalist model of the past have much in common.

There is no standard blueprint for the way in which such a vision can be reached in practice. This is a key factor to consider in thinking about how the medical home concept might impact the future of U.S. primary care. The respected accrediting body, the National Committee for Quality Assurance (NCQA), has developed a detailed array of checklist-based criteria and metrics for determining whether or not practices fulfill the medical home ideal. This checklist aims to become the gold standard against which medical home practices are assessed and measured. But even this attempt at grounding the medical home ideal in everyday primary care practice does not tell PCPs or their places of employment how to get it all done. And getting it done in a way that fulfills the medical home ideal will be extremely difficult within the context of a primary care business model that favors treating patients as customers, pays PCPs almost exclusively to do quick face-to-face visits and not much else, and gets PCPs to give up work that is more time consuming and complex in order to focus on generating patient volume.

The larger health care delivery context is what makes primary care leaders interviewed about the medical home model believe it is not the savior for primary care.

> One of the concerns I have is that we might want to hang the success of the medical home endeavor on total system cost savings, and I think to be fair and honest there has to be some measure of the types of cost drivers that the medical home could have some control over. Because I feel that they're not very big. The cost drivers the medical home can fix are not very big in comparison to systemwide drivers like fee-for-service medicine, imaging, and pharmacy costs. So it's not a panacea for controlling costs in the system. (Bart, family physician and primary care professional association leader)

> .　.　.

> I think there's going to be a lot of other new changes to rebalance the equation. It's not just going to be a lot of new money for medical homes. There needs to be an acknowledgment that with better primary care, there's less specialty utilization, less hospitalizations, less duplication of hospital tests. (Skip, PCP and health plan manager)

Those interviewed about the medical home felt it was a "calculated reach" by health care stakeholders desperate to balance cost and quality in the system. Although conveying optimism about the ability of this approach to be embraced by payers, the medical profession, and patients, there was palpable anxiety about its sustainability in the event it did not produce tangible cost savings. For example, Larry is a practicing internist and medical administrator for a large primary care network that serves suburban and rural areas. He wants the concept to be accepted, but has serious doubts.

> The ethos of medicine in the United States is quick fixes and procedural medicine. And our population is no healthier by pursuing this ethos. But there are some strong lobbies out there that will want to protect this existing system. They will fight to prevent more money from shifting

over into primary care. The other thing is that the culture in the U.S. is autonomy, from the patient's perspective. For the medical home to be perceived as something other than the gatekeeper model we had in managed care will be hard. I find it impossible to believe that the insurance companies are going to give primary care higher reimbursement without seeing some real cost savings in the end. And those cost savings can be speculated on, but it's only after they see diminishing claims for cardiac catheterizations, dermatology visits, plastic surgery visits, cardiology visits, allergist visits, and so on that they're going to say, "Oh, this model does save money," and then they'll be willing to invest in it more. But that means primary care docs are going to have to act as gatekeepers. No one uses that term but the concept is there. (Larry, internist and medical director)

In fundamental ways, the medical home idea is old wine in new skins. Various parts of it have been tried and tested already in U.S. health care. A quick Medline or Google Scholar search on the terms "care coordination" and "case management" bring up thousands of decades-old articles dealing with these topics. These terms were at the heart of the managed care reforms tested during the 1990s. Medical home proponents argue that things were different then because the financing model of managed care (capitation) was not an appropriate model for getting PCPs to either coordinate or manage care in a high-quality manner. Capitation involves the payment to PCPs of up-front dollars on a regular basis to physicians to manage patient care. The implicit incentive working on PCPs under capitation was to control utilization (read: not see patients in the office) in order to keep more of the additional dollars provided to them. Reimbursement for face-to-face office visits under a capitated system would be a low dollar amount or nonexistent, with PCPs expected to earn profit for their practice in significant part from the capitated dollars they received for each patient in the practice.

To me, the first attempt at implementing the concept of the medical home was an offshoot of the managed care era where if you give primary responsibility to primary care physicians and you put them in charge of the management of the patient, and you give them some financial support for that activity, then good things will happen. And I still think that is fundamentally the core concept of the medical home, that most folks are trying to get to, implementing it in one fashion or another. Of course, the failure of managed care to facilitate that process was that capitation in and of itself is a very poor way of creating the right incentive for the physician to do the right things for patients. (Donald, national quality improvement organization leader)

. . .

I think the gatekeeper concept was different in that it was designed as a gate or block to the system. Trying to purchase care at the lowest reasonable amount, allocating referral services appropriately. I see care coordination under the medical home model being different. I see it as being driven by the quality outcome, the end result. I don't think we're saying we're doing this to block the number of services the patient is getting, or to automatically save money, which is what I think the gatekeeper system was designed to do. This is designed to get the highest-quality care in the most efficient way because it's coordinated. (Liz, primary care professional association leader)

. . .

The concept of a central hub or medical home for all patients is in both the model now and the managed care model from a decade ago. Unfortunately, in the managed care model, it got usurped or modified and became sort of a financial model where the practices were put at risk and the motivations to improve care were not there. (Trevor, family physician and medical home leader)

As for the quality principle inherent in the medical home model, a "quality movement" has been going on in the United States for at least a decade, since publication of the Institute of Medicine's seminal "To Err Is Human" report.[2] This report highlighted significant patient safety problems within the U.S. health care system. It called for an industrywide approach to improving quality across hospitals, physician practices, and other health care delivery settings. In the past decade, major efforts have been undertaken to improve quality in U.S. health care delivery, particularly in the ambulatory (primary) care setting. The results have been less than encouraging. Some quality improvements designed to reduce medical errors have facilitated new types of errors, some improvements have not been implemented completely, and high rates of a variety of different types of errors still occur in health care.[3]

Another medical home principle, the use of evidence-based medicine, has been legitimized through the presence of accrediting bodies such as the NCQA, which possess long lists of standards that health plans must adhere to in providing care, as well as through the use by physicians of standardized care guidelines. The "chronic care model" already widely accepted as the goal for how physicians should implement chronic disease management, mirrors the clinically focused components of the medical home.[4]

The medical home principles put forth now are neither novel nor transformative in and of themselves. Yet, from the constellation of different stakeholders pushing this concept, which include large national employers, all the major primary care physician associations, state and federal governments, and large foundations, the medical home idea is one whose time has come in terms of integrating these principles simultaneously into primary care practice. Venture capital from these stakeholders, as well as heaping doses of ideological fervor have been poured into pilot projects across the country implementing medical home approaches.[5] And while current evidence on the effectiveness of this model when implemented in its entirety within large practice settings remains limited, proponents hope that evidence will be gained as practices are motivated and equipped to implement the model's various components.

Factors Making the Difference between Fad and Phenomenon

Those interviewed in this study, leaders of organizations at the forefront of this movement, were worried that the medical home concept would end up as another passing fad.

> We're in the middle of a hype cycle with this. It's been overhyped beyond its potential reward, unfortunately. I think we have a limited period of time, I say like 12–18 months, to show it produces or it will be history. I believe that. (Bart, family physician and primary care professional association leader)
>
> . . .
>
> I think there will be a two- or three-year run, like most things in health care, where the health plans and some big employers and the government will help get all this started. Then, as in any business, we're making the initial investment and we'll need to see something. If practices follow through on the commitment and we begin to see evidence of improved quality and some reduction in costs, then I think it will go on from there. If, on the other hand, some early adopters play with it for a while and then the whole thing fizzles, as many other things have in the past, then the financial support won't continue. (Skip, PCP and health plan manager)
>
> . . .
>
> This is a monster in some ways. In a very positive and affectionate way, but the gathering momentum is incredible. The professional societies [in primary care] have worked very closely together. We've always said from day one this is a model that has to be validated to show it

works. We think it will work. But, you know what, this is something we want studied in a credible way. And we're excited about the attention it's getting, but we're also concerned that it will be undermined by well-placed, perhaps, but poorly designed interventions or, in some cases, entrepreneurs going out there and using the name if not the concept and not creating the model that is envisioned. (Bob, internist and primary care professional association leader)

. . .

I'm nervous that if we can't demonstrate the ease of transition of practices to achieve the patient-centered medical home standards that it's not going to go anywhere. And then we've just gone that much further down the road without figuring out how we are going to sustain primary care medicine. (Liz, primary care professional association leader)

These individuals also worried about the varied way in which stakeholders such as employers, physicians, and insurers thought about the medical home concept. Although the general principles were accepted by all, it was the different motivations for buying into these principles that interviewees worried would prevent the model from improving primary care on a sustained basis.

Part of the problem right now is that you have a lot of disparity in the approach to the concept. Policy makers see it as a way to help achieve universal coverage. Others see it as a way to enhance the practice of primary care. I think a lot of payers see it as a way to implement pay-for-performance reimbursement models that would help limit or reign in their costs. I think patient advocates see it as a way to get patients involved more aggressively in making health care decisions and acquiring health care resources and information on a more regular basis. I think a lot of other providers in health care like hospitals and clinics see it as a way to enhance their access to additional funding for primary care. So, in order to move the concept along, we need someone to take leadership in getting a unified definition. People are jumping onboard right now without any clear consensus of what a medical home really is.

There is something really appealing about the concept. And it is appealing because the system is so broken right now, so dysfunctional, that people are grabbing at anything that looks like a decent alternative. At its very basic level of understanding, people see that the medical home concept has the potential to achieve a variety of things they think are important given the condition of the current environment that we live in.

Again, though, this is not an industry that can change en masse because no single player has market dominance. The power and influence in health care is so broadly dispersed that even if you had one single model everyone agreed on, it would be hard to implement because you have so many different players with different objectives of their own. That's the concern I have. That even as we refine the definition, it will be hard to get there. (Garrett, primary care professional association leader)

Medical home leaders gave pause in speaking about if or how the medical home concept might help to "save" primary care.

If this [the medical home concept] is all done right, then a primary care practitioner's job will be more satisfying and their income will, in the best-case scenario, go up by 50 percent. But even then they are still making one-third what a pathologist or anesthesiologist or a dermatologist makes. So, unless other things are done around all that, it's unsustainable. New grads with hefty debts just won't go into primary care no matter how much fun they hear it is. (Skip, PCP and health plan manager)

Three key components are normally identified as critical to advancing the medical home concept. The first is added payment for PCP care coordination or case management. The second is a minimum level of electronic information system capability within every PCP office practice. The final component is serious efforts within all PCP practices to transform how existing work and patient care are performed, creating extra capacity to assume medical home duties in the process. The underlying premise of paying extra for medical-home-type care is that such care will likely not occur unless PCPs get paid new dollars for it. Given a present business model that rewards large numbers of brief, face-to-face patient visits in a given day, things like care coordination and virtual doctor-patient visits through e-mail, for example, will not occur unless new reimbursement for them is injected into the system.

Between Medicare and RBRVS payment systems, primary care has been undermined for a decade or more.[6] That's the root cause, if you will, of the problem in primary care. Primary care docs are running a low-margin business in the sense that their expenses are the highest for the services they need to provide compared to a surgeon who might have one person in the office while they're off at the hospital making money. So it's a high overhead business in primary care and the reimbursement system has not followed that along. And one of the things the medical home approach could provide is to begin to restructure the payment system to pay primary care in a different way than we pay limited care specialists. It's not just a question of jacking up the fees for specific primary care services, it's really changing what you're buying and how you buy it in primary care. (Bart, family physician and primary care professional association leader)

For the information technology (IT) component of the medical home, the idea is that using IT in a practice enhances population-based care management, produces work efficiencies and greater accountability, and allows for innovative forms of patient access to care.

There's a two-pronged strategy with the medical home. One is trying to reshape the payment environment around some kind of a care management fee or capitated payment so that it acknowledges the fact that much of the capability we need to put into these practices is fixed overhead costs, they're not variable costs. They're infrastructure. On the other hand, if we could flip a switch tomorrow and make that payment happen, most of the practices would not have the ability to take advantage of those enhanced payments. So we need to get people ready for this new way they would get paid. Using registries for chronic illness, tracking labs and referrals, electronic health records, e-mail with patients, patient portals, advanced patient self-management support, these are all capabilities the PCPs need to have. (Bart, family physician and primary care professional association leader)

But it is the third component, full-scale transformation of how work and patient care are performed, that is particularly relevant given the findings of the present study and the business model surrounding PCPs. Medical home proponents felt strongly that added payment for things like care coordination and greater implementation of information technology in a practice would not by themselves produce lasting change, nor guarantee fulfillment of the medical home ideal. The ideal would be realized only when PCPs and their practices recognized the need to review how they structured their everyday work, committed themselves to reducing waste, and placed greater emphasis on the patient as consumer.

In this way, primary care work would need to be reinvented for the medical home model to reach its potential. PCPs would have to change how they thought about their roles as workers, increase their reliance on support staff, become team players, interact in a certain manner with patients, and find ways to alleviate the pressures of seeing patients in the office one after another. Otherwise, the medical home would end up simply being extra payment for tasks done inconsistently across primary care practices—tasks that could easily end once the extra payment stopped or decreased.

> For lots of reasons, I think it may not be a fad. But having said that, if the focus is not on the entire reinvention of primary care around this model and instead is just a better way to do pay-for-performance or a better way to do chronic disease management, which in many markets is how it is starting to get dumbed down to, it will fail. And it will be just another fad. So it's an interesting time, as the insurance companies and large employers are becoming more of a driver to this process, it's becoming more around what saves them money, which is different from how you reinvent primary care for the sake of a patient. I think that's the risky time we're in right now. (Trevor, family physician and medical home leader)
>
> . . .
>
> From my perspective, this is about practice transformation. If you're going to transform the practice, it's got to be for all patients and all pay-ers and all systems. If you're going to adopt patient registries to examine ten quality measures, you've got to be able to transform your practice to look at all of your quality measures or you won't be able to find the ten. So it's helping and assisting the practices with some of the basic tools that they're going to need to change the practice of medicine the way they account for their time, the way they bill, and the way they evaluate that the care they give is effective. And I don't think doctors have done the last thing at all. All of that is going to take a great deal of education and will to change. And if we don't have that will to change, we're going to stumble. (Liz, primary care professional association leader)

Fitting How PCPs Work Now into a
Transformed Medical Home Work Model

Transforming primary care practice to align with the medical home requires greater capacity in a PCP's workday for patient-centered care. This study shows that serious challenges must be overcome in the attempt to create capacity. There is at present little excess time available in the typical primary care prac-tice for doing additional activities. While reorganizing how clinical work is performed or reducing waste in how staff conduct their duties may create more time, it can be assumed that the demands of face-to-face, office-based medicine will not slow down anytime in the near future.

These current demands and the associated PCP adaptations to them has produced workers who value speed, directive interactions with patients, and the minimization of unpredictable complex clinical encounters in the course of a given day. This was seen in how PCPs talked about their workdays, particularly in how they structured patient interactions. The need to see high numbers of patients made them hesitant to engage patients in a way they could not predict or proactively control. It also made them reluctant to free up any time in their workday for anything other than reimbursable office visits.

The medical home model may, over time, lessen the need for some patients to see their physicians in person because of increased use of electronic communication, better triaging of complaints, and better self-management of diseases, which keeps people out of the office. However, PCPs are still almost exclusively reimbursed for their services on the basis of the face-to-face office visit. This is not expected to change in the near future. The reimbursement models for medical home implementation are additive and complementary at present, small in their dollar amounts, and not substitutes for the traditional retrospective, fee-for-service office encounter. PCPs cannot earn their living today by focusing on medical home reimbursement. They must see patients in the office, one after another.

The need for speed and predictability are paramount. If these two qualities help generate the primary source of a PCP's income, it is fair to ask how receptive the typical PCP is on an everyday basis to slowing down, if only temporarily, to engage the unpredictability and lesser compensated activities inherent in medical home components. These components include increased patient-centered communication, serving as a "real time" consultant for others in the practice, developing and updating comprehensive care plans for patients, and allowing patient access to their expertise through nontraditional means such as e-mail. It cannot nor should it be expected that a decade or more of forcing PCPs to practice in an assembly-line-like manner provides an immediately favorable environment for getting practices to innovate in ways that promote new types of patient access goals. As this study demonstrates, PCP mindsets are attuned to the demands of high-volume medicine. Many now function best in a highly transactional workday where repetition reaps financial benefits.

Greater capacity for engaging in patient-centered activities that do not involve face-to-face office visits could also arise from PCPs making better use of their nonphysician support staff. In this way, PCPs would shift more of their traditional office visit schedule to NPs and PAs, or allow their nursing staff to assume duties that involve patient communication and care coordination. The medical home leaders interviewed felt that how such staff was used currently by PCPs would have to change moving forward.

> Physicians in general have not been trained to work as a team. I've talked with a lot of physicians who say, "I don't really want to give up things, because it feels like I'm giving up control." I understand that. But what happens is in a lot of these practices, they don't let people practice to the level of their licensure. And what happens is those people get dissatisfied because you have nurses doing little more than bringing patients back into the exam room and taking basic information like vital signs. This is a huge challenge. You can't just throw people together and expect them to play nice. (Bob, internist and primary care professional association leader)

> . . .

> The way medicine is practiced right now is very far away from being a true team approach to care. One of the hearts of the medical home is a team approach to care where everyone in the office that touches the patient at all has a role and takes a collective responsibility for the quality and cost of care. And I don't mean the old idea of "team" where you have a bunch of people working on the patient and they don't talk to each other. What I'm talking about is the microsystem team from the receptionist to the nurse practitioner to the doc to the billing clerk—all meet regularly to discuss roles, responsibilities, and handoffs. (Bart, family physician and primary care professional association leader)

Bart and several others also highlighted the physician's inherent need to control the patient care process, and how this need could undermine a team-based approach to care. He talked about how many PCPs often interpreted new demands on their practice or new innovations in patient care as responsibilities that fell squarely on their shoulders. This prevented them from seeing the potential value in using staff such as NPs and PAs to facilitate their work. Consistent with Bob's take on how PCPs used these staff in the practice, other PCPs described the role of nonphysician clinical in terms of substitute labor that helped primary care practices see more patients and earn greater profit per patient, because these providers were paid less than physicians. PCPs believed that NPs and PAs could handle a significant portion of the routine care that flowed through the practice each day. However, for medical home implementation, the real question is whether PCPs can engage these types of providers in a care partnership rather than as substitute labor.

For example, could PCPs truly serve as consultants for NPs and PAs as the latter took care of increasingly complex patient conditions, or would PCPs feel the need to see these types of patients exclusively, maintaining a firewall between their own skills and those they felt NPs and PAs possessed? Could PCPs give up some decision-making control and allow their nonphysician providers to assume a wider scope of authority over direct clinical care and care management? To work more independently on the kinds of activities embedded in the medical home approach, NPs and PAs would need greater autonomy.

The PCPs in this study largely left their NPs and PAs alone to practice independently on the routine cases. The sense gleaned from the data was that PCPs wanted these staff to practice independently, without a lot of physician consultation. But determining the tipping point between how much control PCPs could give up to NPs and PAs without feeling competitive with them is difficult. In addition, medical home transformation would mean a higher and possibly more inefficient level of "real-time" interaction occurring between the two work groups, especially if PCPs wanted to have strong oversight over these providers. If PCPs saw this dynamic as something that slowed down their own workday and their ability to get efficiently through a schedule full of office visits, it would be less embraced. And PCPs might still perceive many activities as easier to do themselves than allowing NPs and PAs to do them, with the PCP in a consultant role.

Similarly, if NPs and PAs were expected to take part in medical home activities that involved less of the traditional face-to-face patient care, how would PCPs adapt to that reality? If still viewed as substitute labor, PCPs would be hard pressed to "waste" the time of PAs and NPs on patient activities that either generated modest revenue for the practice, or undermined the practice's ability to maximize the number of patients in the office each day. For example, each block of fifteen minutes an NP or PA spends educating patients, examining patient registry information to identify high-risk patients or quality breakdowns in the practice, or reviewing care plans for needed patient interventions is one less reimbursable visit. In this sense, the willingness of primary care practices to organize staff into integrated care teams or allow the cultivation of new staff roles depends on significant dollars made available for these activities and, in turn, PCPs adapting to a way of thinking that such activities have more value to the practice than face-to-face visits.

As to nurses, it was clear from this study that PCPs used them in the manner medical home leaders believed they were used—to help the physician navigate more quickly through face-to-face office visits, enabling greater numbers of patients on the daily schedule. Nursing staff were described by the intervie-wees as assistants that made the PCP workday predictable and allowed them to focus exclusively on the exam-room encounter. But for practice transformation consistent with medical home principles, PCPs would need to embrace their nursing staff as semiautonomous partners and allow them time to provide services such as case management and care coordination.

> Part of this is about primary care docs making better use of their nursing staff. A lot of practices use people like nurses now just to get people in and out of the exam rooms and take vital signs. But these people could be the ones that handle all of the referrals, interact with the pharmacies to do things like prescription refills, communicate with patients by e-mail, educate them and answer their questions. The [big chain drugstores] are making a killing with their nurse clinics. And what I say is I'd rather have that housed within a primary care practice than down at the corner drugstore. (Trevor, family physician and medical home leader)

Yet, within this cloud lay a silver lining. In today's primary care system, most PCPs are accustomed to relying on nurses, NPs, and PAs to help them navigate their workday. If their mindsets around generating revenue solely through face-to-face visits were eased meaningfully, and PCPs were given a chance to readjust to significant new incentives working on them, the present study suggests that PCPs could rely on their staff in new ways that help imple-ment the medical home model. The evidence points less to an issue about a physician's need to control, for example, or some fixed way of thinking about the limits of staff competency to do things like care management. Instead, PCPs think of their clinical support staff as revenue enhancers, and will make the best use of these resources to remain financially stable. Unless the present pri-mary care business model overhauls significantly, with medical home pay-ments becoming a central part of a practice's balance sheet, it is difficult to imagine most PCPs embracing a new type of reliance on this staff.

PCP Values Impacting Medical Home Transformation

The additional PCP capacity needed to help transform practices in a manner consonant with the medical home model may also be found from extending workdays and encouraging PCPs to engage in "virtual" (non-face-to-face) care, with some of this care occurring outside of normal office hours. Study evidence provides less support for the current appeal of this vision of care among the demographic groups that dominate primary care specialties. For example, greater numbers of young PCPs who value primary care as a "decent job" and all that infers may not be willing to transform their workdays into more fluid, boundaryless events they cannot control as easily. These young physicians were not averse to using information technology in their practices. However, the ones in this study valued predictability, flexibility, and time off. Some worked part-time or in several different clinical jobs, and almost all of them pursued a compartmentalized work schedule of "8 to 6" or similar to fulfill these values.

While young PCPs in the study acknowledged the need to do a small portion of work outside of normal hours, the nature of this work is different from that envisioned as part of the medical home model. The "outside" work they reported doing remained voluntary, sporadic, and under their personal control. It did not involve direct communication with patients or other specialists, or the work of direct patient care, as medical home "virtual" care might. Instead, it entailed completing administrative "chores" such as reviewing lab results and blood work, completing visit notes, and reviewing next-day schedules. Their motivation for doing this work after hours was to bring closure to the current day's work and enhance the predictability and efficiency of the next day's office work.

Unless presented in a manner which convinces them that the values of a "decent job" are not compromised by a more intrusive medical home model, the younger PCP cohort might resist engagement in any significant new work outside of normal work hours. This raises an important tension between the practice transformation associated with medical home implementation and the human capital expected to adapt in accordance with it: new ways of delivering primary care must compete directly with a younger PCP mindset that has already made major trade-offs based on the current way primary care is delivered. Young PCPs might not be that interested in formal work expectations outside of the "8 to 6" workday even if they earn additional income from such activities, since for many in this study, once a certain adequate income level was reached salary was less important than lifestyle. In addition, as salaried employees, their desire to earn greater revenue for the practice as a whole will be less than the personal desire for a particular lifestyle.

Similarly, many of the female PCPs interviewed were in primary care in part due to the flexibility it offered them to take on parental roles. They gravitated to a primary care career, and avoided careers in specialties such as surgery, because a key benefit of the former was having greater control over the structure of the workday. Many younger female physicians in the study were challenged with the simultaneous demands of raising young children and workdays that required them to see large numbers of patients. The emphasis on "making your numbers" to be considered a good colleague put some female PCPs under pressure to make sure they did enough office-based direct patient care to be seen as contributing.

Those with younger children had little excess capacity to take on additional work duties. Since many also worked part time, potential continuity-of-care issues arose with their existing patients because they could not always be on-site for these patients when they came into the office. If part of the practice transformation of medical homes involves greater PCP engagement with patients and allows them more access points to physicians outside of the traditional face-to-face visit, does this run counter to how some female PCPs who are raising families might want to structure their jobs? Will these women allow themselves to be more available throughout a workday to NPs and PAs as consultants, even if they may not be on-site in the practice? Given the numbers of women going into primary care, such questions are central to the future viability of a medical home model with primary care physicians at the core.

On the other hand, evidence that female physicians approach patient care differently from their male counterparts, particularly in the communication and process-oriented aspects of the doctor-patient interaction (for example, they spend more time with patients and focus more on their psychosocial contexts), make this demographic group well suited to many medical home components. Spending time with patients, whether in the office or by phone or e-mail, to gather background information and develop care-management plans, may suit their talents and interests well. In addition, the communication skills of female PCPs, proven in the literature and expounded upon in this study, align with the role of a lead consultant who engages in "real time" dialogue with other staff.[7]

Finally, older PCPs in the study who valued face-to-face encounters were less enamored with the physician-to-physician and physician-to-patient communication possibilities offered by modern information technology. They missed getting to know their patients the traditional way, through exam room conversation. It is questionable to assume that these physicians, long socialized within a model of care that involves seeing as well as listening or reading, will embrace new models of care that ask them to engage in virtual or consultant-type care. Older PCPs had adapted begrudgingly to the high-volume model of care by taking some personal advantage of predictable work hours and greater job flexibility, for example. But even the high-volume model allowed them to practice within the framework of the face-to-face visit. It was a faster, less varied workday, but still one in which they maintained familiarity. Much of the medical home care would require adapting to less familiar ways of doing their work.

The PCP View of Patients and How It Aligns
with the Medical Home Model

Another cultural challenge in transforming primary care practice in a manner envisioned by medical home proponents is the potentially dysfunctional ways PCPs may view patients under the current primary care system. The medical home model promotes greater patient-centered care by encouraging primary care practices to meet patient expectations for customer service. Operationally, it calls for less face-to-face contact between patient and physicians using health information technology, nurse triaging, and direct care by nonphysician providers. It also asks PCPs to assume the role of coaches and mentors for patients to achieve greater patient self-management and education.

There is evidence in the study that PCPs view patients currently in ways that are not consistent with embracing the interventions noted above. PCPs saw patients as expecting quicker service and direct communication with them. However, they were less sympathetic toward meeting these expectations because of their own work demands. Ironically, PCPs interpreted patient demands for quicker, direct contact in mostly negative ways. For example, they saw many patients as too impatient in waiting a reasonable period to receive clinical information such as the results of lab tests or blood work, or as seeking immediate attention through a same-day office visit instead of being open to triage over the phone by a nurse.

Once again, these findings are witness to the destructive power of the existing primary care business model on PCP mindsets. Within a high-patient volume, transaction-based model of primary care delivery, overly complex, "high maintenance," or noncompliant patients become distractions derailing an otherwise efficiently planned workday. These types of patients may also be seen by PCPs as unreasonable consumers unwilling to adapt to how PCPs must practice for financial viability. PCPs who must see set numbers of patients in a daily work schedule feel the need to direct and limit communication opportunities in ways patients may not understand. Within the transactional model of care, what is considered reasonable communication or access expectations, such as getting a lab or test result quickly from the doctor's office, or answering patient questions about test results, the PCP may view as unreasonable. If PCPs do not believe that the typical patient empathizes with their work realities, they may be hesitant to reach out and engage those patients enthusiastically.

The one positive observed in the study that bodes well for the medical home approach is the general favorableness with which PCPs saw a more informed patient. While often grumbling about how a more informed patient created higher expectations for a doctor's time and communication, PCPs saw the benefits for patient self-management and compliance that resulted from a better-educated patient. They believed that in some instances it made their jobs easier and more efficient, particularly if the PCP's assessment was consistent with that already gleaned by the patient from sources such as the Internet. The PCPs in this study liked informed patients when it fed into a higher percentage of patients who left their office assured that the PCP's game plan for treatment was correct. In PCP minds, this created a compliant patient who would follow their direction.

The PCP as "Consultant": Ready, Willing, and Able?

The changes made in primary care to support effective implementation of the medical home model also requires the PCP to step away from some types of patient care, for example the basic acute care now comprising large portions of their workdays, and assume an overall consultant-type role in the practice. This consultant role is a transformation in and of itself, since it forces PCPs to think of themselves in the larger role of team leader. It requires them to avoid enacting their roles as high-level assembly-line workers trying to meet productivity targets. Serving as a consultant forces them into the roles of epidemiologists, looking at practice populations and their care patterns, and teachers for the PAs, NPs, and nurses working with them. Again, evidence presented in this study suggests that such new roles are not commensurate with how PCPs currently work and think about themselves.

Although there were exceptions, such as Billy in chapter 5 who was now running his practice as a lead consultant for nonphysician staff and doing clinical work only for complex care, the PCPs interviewed had adapted to the high-volume business model by focusing their skill enhancements on doing the face-to-face patient visit better. They aimed to increase exam room predictability and move through a daily visit schedule with as few interruptions as possible. They also used support staff in ways that served their professional work interests rather than a medical home-type integrated care approach.

Many PCPs in the study talked of their willingness to avoid overengagement in complex patient issues, in part to maintain a semblance of order in getting through their patient visit schedule. The tendency to become quicker "trigger pullers" for referring patients to specialists and a decreased ability to play the role of "detective" in exploring uncertain diagnostic or treatment situations were part of this mindset. In this way, PCPs had adapted to the high-volume business model by accepting a fixed level of complexity in their daily work. Within a compensation system that rewarded numbers of visits as opposed to time spent during those visits, this adaption was not only appropriate, but good for business.

Similarly, giving up hospital medicine was an adaptation forced onto PCPs by the economics of practice. But PCPs in the study felt something valuable was lost in doing so. For older PCPs, long-standing links and decreased emotional connection to patients were the consequences of this shift. For younger PCPs, self-confidence and a reservoir of experiential knowledge evaporated when the hospital was not part of their everyday work life. In both groups, the sense was that something important was missed because of no longer practicing in the hospital. Some older PCPs were less satisfied in their jobs, and lamented weakened ties to patients, while younger PCPs' lack of hospital experience left them with a more limited view of the doctor-patient relationship in primary care. Either way, greater social and emotional distance between PCP and patient resulted from the absence of hospital work.

Given these findings, it is fair to wonder how many PCPs can meet the knowledge and role expectations implicit in being a true "consultant" in the medical home model. For example, as older PCPs retire and take years of hospital work experience with them, will the younger group possess enough experiential knowledge across a range of illnesses and disease processes to function as more than a lower-level consultant? Billy, for example, was a middle-aged PCP who felt entirely comfortable assuming the role of consultant, providing input on patients he did not necessarily know and had not seen. Yet, it was unclear at what point Billy felt less able to serve in that role, and at what point no longer doing hospital work would begin to undermine his clinical knowledge base.

Less hospital work also means less contact with specialists in fields such as cardiology, orthopedics, urology, and gastroenterology. This decreased contact may reduce the level of up-to-date clinical knowledge possessed by PCPs, affecting their ability to be consultants in their practice for some types of patients and conditions. Several PCPs commented on the disadvantages of losing regular contact with specialists. In addition, the PCP workday is now filled with a high percentage of routine care, even in the area of chronic disease management. If, as PCPs suggested, complex patients face quicker referral out of the practice because of the pressures of the twenty-five to thirty visits per day, the reduced complexity and variety of work affects PCP ability to act as care consultants.

A second consideration shaping PCP ability to meet the knowledge and role expectations of the medical home model involves the increasingly central role played by a primary care practice in behavioral medicine. PCPs in this study talked about how this type of medicine was now a significant part of their workday. They were clear about their limited level of comfort and expertise in practicing it. A major component of the PCP consultant role within a medical home model may be around the diagnosis and treatment of behavioral disorders. It is evident from this study that PCPs will be less comfortable working with other clinical staff on these conditions if they have not met the patient, do not know the patient, or are receiving information not through a personally conducted history and physical, but through secondhand information transmission contained in an electronic health record.

If current attention paid to the medical home translates only into PCPs receiving additional compensation for activities such as care management, care coordination, and patient education, it should increase the likelihood that these activities occur for some patients. However, the PCP attitudes and behaviors observed in this study and the larger organizational milieu in which PCPs now find themselves present more barriers than opportunities to transform primary care practice in comprehensive ways consistent with the medical home approach. As a result, the approach may be short-lived, entirely dependent on extra dollars to maintain its viability, and be implemented through a primary care delivery setting that remains largely unchanged from how it looks and performs now within a transactional business model.

When considering the physicians who do primary care work and the business model that has shaped their thinking, it is clear that the transformation desired by medical home proponents cannot be just a structural transformation. A structural transformation involves making payment or technology available so that virtual, consultant, and team-based care is likelier to happen, restructuring work flows to create additional time in the workday for new forms of care, and developing human resource strategies to advance primary care delivery teams. But a cultural transformation among PCPs must also occur to make the new structures perform to their potential. Part of that cultural shift can happen organically over time if the existing financial incentives and practice structures supporting primary care medicine are changed in meaningful ways. This study provides evidence for that hypothesis in how older PCPs, trained and socialized under different financing and delivery structures, had adapted to the current business model.

But if the present business model remains dominant, if PCPs still gain the bulk of their compensation from generating billable office visits, and if the visit demands on PCPs do not lessen, current attitudes and behaviors might remain hardwired into the collective psyche of the primary care physician community. Many PCPs, especially older ones, long for change from the present practice form. But having already gone through one significant adaption, older PCPs may not readily embrace another one, no matter how good it may be for patient care. It is then up to younger PCPs, who may prefer the present way of doing business because that is the system that allows them to construct their lifestyles in the desired manner.

In either case, both younger and older PCPs will need convincing that whatever transformed business model they are asked to work within, if it now involved medical home components, it becomes one that rewards them for spending more time with patients when needed, coordinating and managing all of a patient's care, and cultivating the doctor-patient relationship. If they are not convinced and view the medical home idea as nothing more than extra and temporary reimbursement that is not worth taking advantage of, little of the wholesale practice transformation advocated by medical home proponents will occur.

Chapter 10

No Quick Fix

An Incremental Approach to Helping Primary Care

It is impossible to imagine a return of primary care to the past, before the transactional, high-volume business model dominated. The golden age of primary care, in which the generalist physician held great sway, specialty medicine was not endemic throughout the health care system, and insurers and patients saw the generalist as a complete caregiver, is over. This decline is the result of several developments including advances in medical science and technology, a quality movement that has downplayed the generalist's value, the media's fixation on exotic types of care, public demands for the best, most sophisticated care possible, and insurer willingness to pay for high-priced, technologically driven service delivery.

This study points to another explanation for the decline of primary care and the generalist physician: the decades-long interplay between the current primary care business model and PCP adaptation to that business model. These twin culprits have interacted with each other for at least twenty years, and the deleterious results of that interaction for the field of primary care are readily apparent. These results include, among other things, declining prestige for primary care in the eyes of the medical profession, payers, and patients; continued economic devaluing and skill narrowing of PCP work; new value systems and expectations among PCP cohorts that may not jibe with the medical home concept or patient expectations; and dramatic reductions in the number of U.S. medical students interested in becoming PCPs.

A new golden age for generalist medicine is less plausible given our current health care system. But the future for PCPs and primary care medicine is not bleak. While the work and workers of primary care undergo transformation, the demand rises for primary care services. The growing number of ambulatory care visits made in the United States, rising rates of chronic disease and behavioral disorders, extended life spans mean, and national health reform that emphasizes primary, preventive care will further strain the primary care system.[1] The conditions afflicting most individuals, and costing the system most in terms of money, quality of life, and lives are basic chronic illnesses that do not rely on sophisticated technology, technicians, surgeons, or procedural medicine to identify, prevent, or treat in the less acute stages. They rely on regular contact with the primary care system and a prevention-oriented brand of medicine.

Even with competition from new structures like retail clinics, visits to a traditional primary care practice will not decrease any time soon. First, there is enough demand to satisfy all of these new structures, and at present each structure serves a somewhat different consumer market.[2] Second, the care for many patients at the primary care level grows multifaceted and complex because individuals are less healthy on average. The vast majority of the physician expertise needed for this type of care is found in traditional practice settings, not in retail clinics or urgent care centers. Right now, PCPs are in demand. A national physician recruitment firm reported in a 2008 survey of its physician recruiting trends that they engaged in more recruitment searches for family medicine and internal medicine than any other medical specialty.[3] This trend was similar to one observed in 2007. Salaries offered to family and internal medicine physicians have also increased over the past several years.[4]

The availability and acceptance of alternative providers such as nurse practitioners (NPs) and physician assistants (PAs) will not erode the central role PCPs play in caring for many patients. If the medical home model is implemented in a substantive way, then PCPs will be asked to serve as leaders, direct-care providers, and consultants for much of the complex primary care medicine delivered to sicker patients. In this way, a successful medical home model can reassert the PCP's standing in primary care. But NPs and PAs will carve out their own sphere of independent work given the continued decline in the PCP workforce, shortages of PCPs in underserved areas of the country, and the continued growth of structures such as retail clinics.[5]

Making Primary Care Medicine Matter

The bigger policy question is how to make PCPs and primary care medicine fulfill their potential in a fragmented health care system that needs skilled generalists. It makes sense, given patterns of aging, disease prevalence, and the current costs of care for the U.S. health care system and patients to have primary, preventive care as its backbone. But specialty care now plays that anatomical role for the entire system. We are in the midst of a technological and procedural golden age in U.S. medicine where high-cost acute care has the blessing of payers and patients.

The U.S. health care system will remain a specialty-dominated system, regardless of whether or not approaches like the medical home or the incremental options presented here are tried. The health care industry has gone too far emphasizing high-tech, high-cost specialty medicine to be able to change quickly. Too much money and power are at stake for groups of physicians, hospitals, and other stakeholders to acquiesce to primary care willingly, even if it makes sense. No one appears to want to move the really big money away from specialty care to service delivery that prevents disease and promotes health.

We cannot expect primary care physicians to change this reality in the short run. Their position within medicine presently is too weak to gain the kinds of economic or legislative changes needed that would begin to shift emphasis more toward generalist medicine. Instead, the goal should be to make generalist medicine *worth something* once again to patients, politicians, the medical profession, and insurers. Being worth something in this case is a function of having a recognizable value to the outside world, gaining control over work that feeds into creating that value, and possessing a stable, competent workforce that is motivated to do this valuable work. Right now, the field of primary care faces challenges in all of these areas.

If primary care is to get healthier in the United States, PCPs must get paid more and their business model must change. As this study shows, PCPs have adapted to their business realities in ways that are economically rational but further transform the patient encounter into rushed, impersonal affairs. This transformation of the patient encounter into a customer transaction erodes the public's perception of generalist doctors because it obscures the added value these doctors provide if given the time and incentive to do so. Time-pressured PCPs whom patients cannot know, trust, listen to, and see on a regular basis become indistinguishable from other providers who do not profess so openly to offer these rewards. And when this happens, the perceptual line blurs between what a PCP-led primary care practice might offer over a retail clinic or urgent care center.

In a specialty-dominated delivery system, only major legislative action could shift reimbursement schemes toward primary care in ways that make a difference. The medical home approach might temporarily put tens of thousands of additional dollars annually into each PCP's pocket. But this added reimbursement will not always be available, especially if the cost savings and quality improvements expected by insurers and employers (the stakeholders funding medical home experiments nationally) do not materialize in timely, significant ways.

PCPs will not change overnight the way they now practice simply because they are getting a few extra dollars to do new things. The fact is patients still have to physically come into the PCP's exam room each day for the practice to generate enough revenue to survive, and unless this imperative lessens, everything else—care management, care coordination, virtual patient care—remains subservient to it. The likelihood that fewer individuals will walk through primary care practice doors is slim in the short term, so face-to-face visit reimbursement in primary care must improve, with PCPs getting paid appropriately for conducting longer visits that involve the cognitive medicine necessary for proper prevention, chronic disease management, and behavioral health care.

Besides reimbursement, two additional workplace elements that can enhance the value of primary care in the eyes of patients include better alignment of PCP interests and skill sets with the required care demands now present at the primary care level, and a redistribution of primary care services that apportions different types of primary care medicine to the most cost efficient, timely, and appropriate delivery setting. Existing PCP adaptation to the high-volume model of care has eroded key interpersonal qualities and clinical competencies needed for medical-home-type care. Especially for younger PCPs, the field needs to provide significant education and training in the areas of practice leadership, teamwork, care management, psychosocial or behavioral medicine, and interpersonal communication. Some PCPs may have to learn or relearn what it means to have a continuous, deep patient relationship that calls upon them to be vigilant, proactive overseers of care. The skills that go into making such relationships work are not born into every physician. They also are not presently called upon for use in a business model that rewards brevity of contact.

A case can also be made for looking at the twenty-first century landscape of primary care delivery and redistributing services in ways that recognize the strengths and weaknesses of the various structures and care providers that now exist. For the sake of increasing both the efficiency and overall service capacity within primary care, nonphysician providers and new structures such as retail clinics should be encouraged by physicians, insurers, and state and federal legislatures to assume a central role in the delivery of lower-level primary care. The sheer volume of visit demands placed on traditional primary care offices undermines a practice's ability to deliver complex, personalized care to patients and thus show the richer value of generalist medicine to patients. Already, some hospitals and health care systems have moved strategically to incorporate urgent care centers and retail clinics into their businesses.[6] More are likely to follow. And traditional primary care practices already use NPs and PAs as substitute labor to provide lower-level care, as seen in the present study.

But besides the profit motives underlying these moves, there is an opportunity to ease the strain on traditional primary care practices and PCPs for the exclusive purpose of having the latter provide complex, relationship-oriented primary care medicine in better ways. As long as PCPs see basic acute care, for example, as a key part of their "bread-and-butter" service offerings, they will neglect to innovate around complex care delivery, case management, and care coordination. Even if adequate payment is provided for these activities, the question is whether there is enough extra capacity within traditional primary care settings to assume the full scope of physician-led services called for by a model like the medical home.

Strategic partnerships to enhance the economic and social value of primary care can be made between delivery settings and providers that normally view each other as competition. These partnerships are facilitated by a payment and legislative environment that is committed to putting primary care at the center of a reformed health care system. PCPs and the professional associations to which they belong should not view such partnerships as encroachments on their turf. Instead, it is a survival tactic aimed at shifting some degree of real economic power and prestige back to primary care medicine, no matter which worker or structure delivers that medicine.

There are other worker-focused policy considerations and strategies that might contribute positively to a primary care turnaround. This study provides clues for how to make additional improvements aimed at enhancing the primary care physician workforce that would, when tried together, do several things: heighten the perception of primary care as a complex, varied part of medicine; help attract more bright young doctors to primary care and keep them satisfied; allow generalist physicians to maintain control over key parts of primary care medicine that are in high demand; prepare young PCPs better for practicing today's primary care medicine; and position the field of primary care within the U.S. medical profession and health system in a way that raises its economic and social value. These improvements involve increasing the scope and substance of exposure to primary care work and careers in medical training; rebranding primary care careers to emphasize its lifestyle benefits above all else; and enabling the field of primary care to assert greater control over behavioral health and hospital work.

Increasing the Scope and Substance of
Primary Care Exposure in Medical Training

One PCP in the study commented that medical schools and residency programs often do the right thing ten years or more after the time it should be done, the point being that as a highly bureaucratic institution medical training cannot shift emphasis easily or cheaply. Medical training has let the field of primary care wither away because it has not moved quickly enough to innovate in ways that would inspire more students and young physicians to become primary care physicians. The external focus on "pull" strategies of higher PCP salaries, better working conditions, and a wider scope of complex, stimulating work to resuscitate generalist medicine obscures the many internal "push" strategies that the medical profession, in training its future members, could experiment with to raise the popularity of primary care.

Listening to today's medical students and residents, it is clear that primary care training is in need of a Madison Avenue makeover. The first two years of medical school are fraternity hazings that pit students against one another in an artificial environment of exam after exam, the Pavlovian absorption of textbook facts that will appear on the next test, only to be forgotten once the test is over, and rote memorization of both useful and useless material that crowds out extended learning opportunities. Students fixate on passing the first "step" of the medical licensing board exams, which tests the application of basic science knowledge to medical issues. This exam positions them for competitive residency programs; medical schools fuel fixation on the exam because it is in their best interests to have their students perform well on the boards.

Surveys of trainees going back a decade demonstrate that primary care is viewed by significant numbers of future doctors as less intellectually rigorous and stimulating, and a primary care career as less favored by medical schools and faculty mentors than other specialties.[7] A national survey of over two thousand academic faculty, residents, and medical students showed that primary care work was perceived as requiring less expertise and being less difficult than specialty work, and deemed primary care doctors as less appropriate than specialists to treat even common patient ailments such as back pain and asthma.[8]

Some argue a pervasive culture exists within medical training that looks down on primary care.[9] In the same survey noted above, meaningful percentages of primary care faculty, the individuals who are supposed to be role models for young physicians interested in generalist medicine, also felt that primary care doctors were less prepared than specialists to handle complex care. Perhaps most disturbing was that less than half of one percent of all students and residents surveyed felt that academic faculty encouraged capable trainees to enter a primary care field for their career choice.[10] Students, residents, and young physicians in this study spoke similarly of the negative or ambivalent manner in which medical school faculty, academic medical center physicians, and the prevailing medical school culture viewed primary care careers.

Impressionable students who work hard to get into medical school may not automatically know what type of physician they wish to become. While more may be open to primary care careers at the beginning of their medical training, they pick up quickly on any ambivalence and hostility toward primary care exhibited by their teachers and mentors. This socializes them early to regard primary care as unattractive. The training environment in academic medical centers must acknowledge that it is a significant part of this problem. The fact that it has not done so on a widespread scale, and instead pointed its collective finger at external economic forces that undermine the primary care system, holds back primary care reform.

The essence of a primary care makeover would involve injections of both style and substance into medical training and how primary care is presented to medical students and residents. First and foremost, medical training must address directly the need to change how students and residents gain exposure to primary care work and doctors. To hear medical students describe it, primary care is noticeably absent during the first two years of medical school. Yet, it is during this time when primary care might first attempt to change the perception that it is neither as rigorous nor as appropriate as other specialties to handle a wide spectrum of diseases and care situations. This might also be the time when the larger societal contribution made by primary care medicine, in terms of providing a safety net for the underserved population and compassionate, continuous care for individuals in poor health, as well as personalized care for the middle class, could be highlighted for medical students. Some of them may have strong feelings at this early training stage about the type of public service they wish to provide as physicians.

However, these early years of training, with curricula organized dryly around basic science courses, learning about specific organ systems and disease mechanisms, and debating more exotic patient cases, convinces students that care fragmentation is an appropriate reality, that specialists know better than anyone how to practice real medicine (because they teach most of the curriculum), and that primary care is the first and least competent line of defense in diagnosing and treating illness. The students in this study, from two different medical schools, felt the deck was stacked against primary care from the moment of the first medical school class.

The first two years of medical school must include primary care physicians centrally as teachers, and the primary care perspective must be integrated into as many cases and teachable moments as possible. Faculty should also use primary care teachers and role models to give students heavy doses of training in less exotic but more common clinical responsibilities such as care continuity, chronic disease management, and behavioral healthcare. Having primary care faculty in central teaching roles may not produce vast numbers of students with greater interest in primary care,[11] but doing so sends an important message that the basic science knowledge contained in generalist clinical medicine deserves equal billing with the narrower, compartmentalized knowledge of specialty clinical medicine. It will also allow students greater exposure to the type of medicine PCPs perform, medicine that is more holistic, continuous, and prevention oriented than specialty medicine.

First- and second-year medical students now participate in experiences that allow them to observe how primary care is conducted in community-based settings that offer richer, more varied exposure to primary care work.[12] But it is in the classroom where they see mainly specialists and specialty views on health and illness. It is not enough to add an extra primary care elective course during the students' first two years. It is not enough to provide interested students with the chance to observe primary care physicians in their offices. In fact, these actions may serve only to convince students that generalist medicine is on the periphery of "real" medical training. Instead, as many mainstream courses as feasible, basic science and otherwise, must integrate the generalist perspective during the first two years of medical school.

The importance of primary care faculty role models in getting students interested in a primary care career is identified repeatedly.[13] Yet often students do not see these role models enough in the earliest years of their training. If they do, what they see are overworked clinicians who must play to incentives different from those of the academic researchers and revenue-generating physicians employed by cardiology, surgery, and neurology departments. What they see are individuals who have neither the time nor energy to teach or mentor them, even when they are encouraged to do so, because of the heavy amounts of direct patient care their hospital asks of them.

In addition to academic faculty, medical schools must bring in community-based PCPs to teach and advise students and develop pedagogic models that connect basic science understanding to primary care practice in as many courses as possible. Several practicing PCPs in this study said they would like to get involved more with their local medical school, but it was not financially feasible for them to do so. If medical colleges could innovate with respect to when and how courses are delivered to students, such as scheduling some courses in the evenings or on weekends when community-based PCPs might be able to participate, or perhaps offer more courses in the curriculum online, the "town-gown" dichotomy that treats what happens in academic medical centers as loftier than or detached from community-based practice work might begin to break down.

Making Primary Care Clerkships and
Resident Experiences More Attractive

Medical residency training also must share the blame for turning students and young physicians off to generalist medicine. When one looks at the structure of primary care residency programs, the overwhelming conclusion reached is how misaligned current primary care residency training is relative to what most PCPs end up doing once they practice. For example, almost no PCPs do hospital work anymore, yet all three primary care specialties train their members almost exclusively within the hospital setting.

During years three and four of medical school, and in the residency experience awaiting students after that, it is not the quantity but rather the quality of primary care exposure that must be changed. If hospital clinics and inpatient settings are the main sources of exposure to primary care physicians and their work, then primary care will look unappealing to most rational medical students. Primary care is low on the totem pole in a hospital environment compared to specialty care, giving residents the impression in everyday training settings that primary care is not valued by the system, and that inpatient and episodic acute care is most important.[14] If the majority of primary care role models in residency programs are overworked academic faculty or senior residents who ply their trades daily in an environment where primary care medicine is subservient to specialty medicine, where inpatient care demands the bulk of resources and attention, and where workloads are intense, then a primary care career will look like one that is second rate, frustrating, and less prestigious.

A review of over seventy studies addressing how students get interested in and choose primary care careers concluded that primary care experiences for students that involve community-based, longitudinal care experiences have positive impacts on individuals selecting primary care careers.[15] Surveys also consistently show that students selecting primary care are attracted by opportunities for direct patient care, continuity of care, ongoing patient relationships, clinical variety, and psychosocial medicine.[16] However, most primary care clerkships and residencies still place young physicians in hospital-based clinic environments that cannot provide such experiences. Ironically, it has been pointed out that some attempts in academic settings to increase resident and student exposure to primary care work and careers backfire in providing experiences that reflect poorly on the field as a whole.[17] The voices in this study bear this out. Sarah, the general internist who taught several years in an Ivy League–affiliated medicine residency program, spoke of how unattractive the generalist primary care work experiences were in her program because they overemphasized work in the hospital outpatient clinic where sicker, more noncompliant patients presented in an understaffed, chaotic work environment.

On paper, the goal is to provide residents who staff outpatient clinics with continuity-of-care and disease-management experiences. But the fragmented nature of the medicine residency year, with its various rotations and outpatient care work spread over weeks at a time, made this goal difficult to realize. It also placed the burden on residents to pursue a favorable primary care training experience while working in a surrounding context that provided good reasons not to do it. It is not only internal medicine residency programs that suffer from this problem. The vast majority of pediatric and family medicine residencies are aligned closely with an academic medical center. While their requirements (especially in the field of family practice) call for lengthy training experiences in outpatient care, their patient panels also include significant numbers of the kinds of patients Sarah saw in her everyday work.

Primary care residency programs, when housed in hospital-based ambulatory care departments, do not offer the right balance of primary care experiences that individuals are likely to have once out of training. For example, more PCPs practice in clinical settings that have diverse, middle-class patient bases. These settings are filled with patients who have different health issues, and to varying degrees compared to the limited patient variety seen in the hospital-based clinic. It is logical that a significant portion of primary care student clerkships and residency experiences should take place in community-based, primary care office settings that offer better patient variety and a potentially more relevant primary experience.

But involving private-practice settings in residency training is no easy task. First, as PCPs in this study noted, medical students are a drag on the time of community-based physicians. They slow them down, and, in the midst of a busy workday built on volume, slowdowns are not welcome. These settings are unreceptive to training students and residents given the lack of financial incentives to do so. Medical schools, third-party payers, or a specific governmental program would have to subsidize community-based offices to work with medical students and residents. One source of funds available to some schools could be from endowments. These dollars are often used for new educational and practice initiatives. They could be used to provide partial subsidies to community-based practices for training their young physicians. In addition, public insurance programs could enhance primary care reimbursements for PCPs who show they are actively mentoring students and residents while performing their work.

A second barrier is the loss of cheap physician labor that would result from having primary care residents working in private-practice settings. Residents generate revenue for the hospital at a lower per-patient cost than fully licensed physicians. They also aid in providing charity care with less financial loss to the institution. But just as innovation is occurring outside of academic medical centers, in terms of incorporating less expensive, nonphysician providers into basic primary care delivery, similar changes could be considered for these settings. For example, closer linkages with nursing and physician-assistant training programs, and embracing nonphysician trainees to work alongside primary care residents and faculty who see patients within hospital clinics, might free up residents to pursue private-practice experiences without hurting the hospital's bottom line or commitment to caring for the underserved.

Increasing the scope and substance of primary care exposure in medical training should be a top policy concern of medical schools, primary care professional associations, and state and federal legislatures. This "push" strategy will make it easier for medical students and residents to like and understand primary care medicine. As a result, more members of these target groups would consider the possibility of a primary care career. This strategy will not produce a stampede into primary care, but it will increase the number and quality of candidates that primary care careers can market to and recruit.

Getting *all* students and residents to better appreciate the value and expertise involved in generalist medicine when they are most susceptible to these messages (during their training) would also create a larger number of future physicians who appreciate the need for primary care, value the role of the generalist physician, and support the centrality of primary care within the larger health care system. Having PCPs and specialists who can convey the importance of primary care to patients is a critical step in getting society to understand and value this branch of medicine.

Rebranding the Primary Care Career as Lifestyle-Focused

A primary care makeover should also focus on marketing the field as providing the best, most family supportive lifestyle of all medical specialties for the young physician. This is a risk, particularly if an innovation such as the medical home model places greater work demands on PCPs, but the field of primary care has few competitive advantages left to advertise compared to other specialties. Attempting to market primary care careers as providing similar excitement or value as surgery, or as having a knowledge base equal in complexity to other specialties, whether true or not, is an ineffective tactic. First, there are enough counterarguments other specialties can make about the excitement, value, and knowledge questions that young physicians are apt to listen to. Second, these arguments still do not touch upon the main factor considered by medical students and residents when making particular specialty choices. Since "controllable lifestyle" and all that implies is now that factor, there are compelling messages to be crafted about primary care work and careers in this regard that should appeal to meaningful numbers of these two groups.[18]

The reality of a primary care career where people pursue satisfied, well-balanced lives while earning a decent income is simply not sold enough to the younger cohort of medical students and residents. Currently, popular specialties like hospital and emergency medicine are sold that way, with their overt emphasis on shift work, lots of time off, time off that is consecutive, and few hassles once the doctor leaves the hospital at the end of his or her shift. If primary care could promote such lifestyle advantages and heighten these positive perceptions with additional changes in its job structures and employment alternatives, it is reasonable to expect that additional medical students would choose primary care. With PCP salaries also increasing as a result of greater marketplace demand, it would help stem the rapidly declining number of doctors who now choose general primary care as a career.

Take as an example the growing cohort of female medical students now interested in primary care careers. Marketing pediatrics, family medicine, or general internal medicine as careers that allow women physicians to practice the type of medicine (with a focus, for example, on psychosocial aspects of care) they prefer, or as jobs in which they can take time off or work part time without professional resentment, could result in attracting more of the best and brightest female medical students to primary care. With many medical specialties still presenting as male-dominated, hostile work environments for women, primary care careers have a competitive advantage with a female demographic that remains untapped.

This lifestyle-focused pitch would be accompanied by the embracing of job structures and employment arrangements that support the field. For instance, more jobs that are part time or take advantage of job sharing arrangements among clinicians could appeal to male and female PCPs who value time off for whatever personal reasons. Part-time clinical positions that structure hours in the middle of the workday could appeal to female PCPs who are young mothers.

This would allow them to spend time with their children in the morning, and then reconnect with them in the afternoon. On the other hand, single PCPs or those without children may opt for a different part-time job structure, one that enables them to work long hours on consecutive days but then get multiple days off in a row, similar to the hospitalist or emergency medicine employment model.

Job sharing for a physician sounds odd at first, because we usually think of arrangements such as these for less-skilled labor. However, the concept could be implemented in a way that is satisfying for the patient, practice, and PCP. If practice expectations for productivity and quality of care were placed on groups of two or three PCPs within a practice who wished to work part time and share compensation based on their individual contributions to team performance, this strategy might enhance individual performance among part-time PCPs while alleviating the pressures placed on each individual to produce in the same manner as the full-time PCP. Patients might accept, if it was made clear to them in advance, the idea that they would have two or three PCPs assigned as their primary care physician "team," and that these physicians would work in a partnership to provide high-quality care and improved access.

Structurally, the continued evolution of traditional primary care practices toward larger size is consistent with facilitating lifestyle-focused employment strategies. Smaller free-standing primary care practices, rapidly disappearing in many areas of the country, would have to be replaced by larger networks of practices that assume the business responsibilities for PCPs, free them to practice medicine, spread the fixed costs of running a practice over a larger number of individuals, and provide a larger pool of PCPs who can negotiate work and free time among themselves. Much as the PCPs in this study saw the value of practicing in a corporate model of employment, younger students and residents would see that taking a primary care job in such settings allows them different ways of maintaining the lifestyle they want. Strength exists in numbers, and PCPs who could negotiate their everyday work responsibilities and personal benefits within a practice setting that has diverse work options available would produce a larger pool of satisfied PCPs.

Two challenges exist to promoting the lifestyle advantages of primary care careers. First, other changes now on the primary care radar screen would need to be examined for how they align with the lifestyle strategy. Chief among these changes is the medical home approach being explored for primary care practices. As discussed in the previous chapter, the medical home model potentially increases the diversity and unpredictability of patient care responsibilities placed on the PCP, which might undermine expectations around lifestyle that younger PCPs value. It may also undermine attempts at creative job restructuring to support enhanced lifestyle, since practices may have little spare capacity to move away from employment models that make maximum use of the physicians on their payroll.

The second major challenge is the possibility that the lifestyle advantages marketed to young physicians and students, combined with changes in job structures to accommodate those advantages, further entrenches the negative perception of primary care as a field that is less challenging and prestigious than other medical specialties. Given what is already a reduced scope of work in primary care, and the perception among many students and residents that primary care consists of a less intellectually rigorous set of specialties, the argument is that primary care cannot afford to have anything associated with it that advances the "consolation career prize" belief in the younger cohort.

This is a risk worth taking. Reversing current negative perceptions about the intellectual content and rigor of generalist medicine among some students and residents is a long-term, difficult, and perhaps unnecessary endeavor, one that other medical specialties will take on and defeat directly. The reality is that the field of primary care should not lose any more students and residents to other careers because of greater perceptions of it as less rigorous or stimulating, making the risk negligible. After all, when only twenty-four of over 1,100 fourth-year medical students recently surveyed across eleven different medical schools say they are becoming generalists, there are few individuals left to lose.[19] Rather, the idea behind the lifestyle strategy is to poach additional students and trainees who may initially express interest in specialties such as hospital or emergency medicine because of favorable lifestyle possibilities, but could also consider a general primary care career given an equally compelling lifestyle argument.

Acquiring Greater Control over Select Domains of Care

Two key opportunities exist for primary care practitioners to expand their scope of work. This expansion is necessary to counteract the reductions in scope that have occurred over the past several decades, in particular the loss of procedural work and hospital medicine. First, the field of primary care can attempt to exert greater occupational control over the work of behavioral health care, due to a perfect-storm combination involving high rates of mental health diagnoses in the general population, the reality that large numbers of these diagnoses first present and get treated in primary care offices, and shortages of traditional mental health clinicians, especially for children and the elderly.

The primary care system acts as the main gateway into the health care system for behavioral health patients, with the large majority of psychotropic medications taken by these patients prescribed and managed in primary care offices. The ability to gain greater control over this work for primary care specialties would, if successful, enhance the prestige of generalist medicine in the public's eyes, formally recognize the new variety associated with primary care work that includes complex psychosocial conditions, and emphasize to insurers the importance of cognitive medicine in the generalist physician's everyday work.

Currently, the provision of mental health services in primary care settings is not reimbursed or recognized adequately. PCPs provide behavioral health care in an environment that does not allow them to bill appropriately for such services, making the services nonvalued parts (from an economic perspective) of an already hectic workday. A recent government report outlined significant barriers to the provision of mental health services in primary care. Chief among these were the inability of PCPs to bill solely for mental health services provided, existing rules that disallow PCPs from billing for physical and mental health services in the same patient visit, lack of reimbursement for collaborative care and case management for mental health services, and lack of reimbursement for mental health screening and prevention in primary care settings.[20] These payment limitations enhance the chances for suboptimal behavioral health care in primary care settings. At the least, they produce frustrated PCPs who grow dissatisfied when presented with too many mental health diagnoses in a given workday, and who feel they cannot provide adequate care for these diagnoses. That frustration was evident in this study.

What would it take for primary care specialties to advance their occupational claims on behavioral health work? The reimbursement issue is obvious, and any significant health care reform nationally should include in it reimbursement opportunities for primary care offices to prevent, diagnose, and treat mental health conditions. A second key element involves appropriate training for PCPs in student clerkships and residency programs that would prepare them to perform this work competently. Primary care residents and residency program directors want more training in their programs that deal with the full scope of mental health service provision, from preliminary interviewing to psychopharmacology.[21] One survey of fifty-four primary care internal medicine residency directors identified an average of only seventy hours of clinical training devoted to psychiatric training over a three-year residency period.[22] This represents less than two weeks of a three-year residency for work that makes up a significant portion of a PCP's workday once he or she is in practice.

The medical home model can also further PCPs' claim on behavioral health work. On paper, this model promotes innovative care partnerships that could be applied to mental health care. From the PCP perspective, strengthening linkages with psychologists and social workers would enhance their legitimacy to practice this type of medicine. For psychologists and social workers, partnering with PCPs offers a prestige bump through closer connection with prescribing clinicians and greater direct contact with patients in a primary care setting. Most importantly, such a partnership would likely produce better integrated care for patients whose psychological and somatic conditions often interact with each other.

A second opportunity for an expansion of primary care work involves reconnecting to the world of hospital medicine. Early research shows the benefits of using hospitalists to decrease inpatient lengths of stay while maintaining quality of care.[23] But there is concern that the connection between hospitalists and office-based PCPs must improve to assure that timely, accurate information gets communicated to the primary care setting once a patient is out of the hospital, and also to the hospitalist at the time of patient admission.[24] The gaps in care continuity that might occur through use of a hospitalist model, resulting from service fragmentation, communication breakdowns, and the lack of in-depth patient knowledge on the part of the hospitalist represent opportunities for PCPs and their professional associations to pursue tighter linkages between office and hospital-based care.[25]

Opportunities for greater collaboration between hospitalists and PCPs are possible through the medical home approach and increased use of health information technology. By giving incentives to PCPs to be care coordinators, the medical home model should give them an appropriate, compensated rationale to spend additional time communicating with hospitalist colleagues when their patients are hospitalized, visit their patients more in the hospital, and pursue work-related innovations that allow them to better control the handoffs that occur when patients are admitted to and discharged from the hospital. However, the added reimbursement for these coordination activities must still compare in economic value to the reimbursement gleaned from the face-to-face office visits PCPs participate in at the expense of hospital medicine.

Through greater use of electronic health records and communication technology linking primary care practices with the hospital environment in real time, PCPs would enhance their ability to engage in ongoing decision making for their hospitalized patients, provide a valuable source of patient information to hospitalists, and keep up to date on advances in different specialty fields. The medical home and health information technology enhancements now being experimented with in primary care settings should help reposition the office-based PCP as the clinician who oversees the entire scope of care for patients, including when patients are in the hospital. They do not have to make every inpatient decision, nor do they have to go to the hospital every day. But by disassociating themselves so completely from hospital work, their decision-making role has been diminished or eliminated altogether.

Besides these enhancements, there is value for primary care practices, particularly larger ones, to participate directly in the care of their hospitalized patients as a "loss leader" service, one in which profit is not earned through the specific activity yet has a positive impact on other revenue-producing services in the practice. This might mean that several office-based PCPs employed by larger practices continue to see hospitalized patients for a portion of their weekly work time, or the practice employs its own hospitalists and does not contract with an independent hospitalist service or company to care for its patients, which has become popular. The additional goodwill gained from patients toward PCPs and primary care practices that retain hospital care in-house can enhance patient satisfaction, patient loyalty to the practice, and trust toward the PCP. Through a medical home approach, it could also allow PCPs to manage their most expensive, complex patients efficiently within a care management payment mechanism that rewards reduced hospitalizations and serious illness.

These modest suggestions for getting primary care medicine to have a stable workforce, greater value within and outside of the medical profession, and the ability to meet the clinical and emotional demands patients make on PCPs when needing care require greater public recognition of what primary care medicine can do. But it will take a generation before such recognition is once again widespread, even if we seriously start that process now. We have been raised in a health care system that does not push us to stay healthy, prefers waiting until we get sick to care for us, and will not pay or innovate around basic acute care and preventive medicine. As a result, while we use and rely on generalist medicine, we take for granted how, when done right, it improves the quality of our lives, reduces our dependency on high-cost medicine, and keeps us out of the physician's office. In the meantime, we can take the small but important steps needed to create a primary care infrastructure that is ready, able, and willing to perform the kind of generalist medicine an aging population will need, and a younger population that is left to pay off the financial tab of the health system we now have will want.

How the Study Was Conducted

Interviews for the study were conducted between summer 2007 and fall 2008. The interview sample consisted of eighty-eight different primary care physicians and two nonphysician primary care leaders. The main purpose of the study was to describe, from the primary care physicians' point of view, their careers, everyday challenges, work experiences, and adaptations as a group of professionals working within an evolving model of service delivery. The sociological focus on PCPs, their work, and how they have adapted is warranted because of a lack of systematic information in the literature about how this occupational group has navigated the business realities imposed on them. It provides a representation of the world both as it exists and is perceived by the physicians as workers.

The study sought to place into its proper social, economic, and psychological contexts the current challenges the field of primary care faces. These contexts interact to shape where primary care is likely headed as a field. How PCPs think about the manner in which they have adapted to the economic realities of their jobs, for example, has implications for future adaptations on their part. Their specific adaptations produce the experiential base upon which further career and job risks are contemplated. In addition, what younger, female, or immigrant PCPs value in their careers or jobs generally influences what the field of primary care will embrace or reject in terms of future work and employment.

The present study was qualitative in nature. The larger analytic aim of the rich description presented here is to inform the bigger-picture discussion around the transformation of primary care medicine in the United States. The ninety unique individuals participating in this study are not a trivial number of people with whom to spend an hour or more on average conversing in depth. By letting PCPs from different backgrounds and contexts give their stories and perspectives, the study did not impose a preordained interpretative lens but rather allowed insights to emerge organically from the data.

The qualitative approach is open to criticisms of idiosyncratic sampling, analytic bias, and nongeneralizability. However, several steps were taken in the research design to increase the "believability" of the findings, a key litmus test for all qualitative research. First, the interviews were spread out over two major time periods to provide an opportunity for preliminary analysis that could feed into later interviews. This process of "theoretical sampling"[1] allowed meaningful findings emerging through early data collection to assume a more prominent focus in subsequent data collection. It is based on the assumption that such findings represent potentially central insights that hold greater descriptive or explanatory power for the dataset as a whole. The first time period for data collection and analysis was summer to fall 2007. Sixty-five interviews were conducted during this time period. These interviews were analyzed during fall and winter 2007–2008, and thirty additional interviews were conducted between December 2007 and October 2008. Two separate interviews were conducted with five of the ninety PCPs, bringing the total number of interviews in the study to ninety-five.

Second, the interview sample was selected purposively based on several demographic criteria that are particularly relevant to the primary care work and career experience in the early twenty-first century. Groups of participants were randomly chosen that fit within each of these desired criteria (see Table 2). The criteria included the following:

- PCPs of different ages and career stages—early, middle, later
- Male and female PCPs with or without children
- PCPs across all three primary care specialties—pediatrics, internal medicine, and family medicine
- PCPs employed in different clinical settings—academic practices, suburban practices serving healthier populations, and clinics serving largely poorer and sicker populations
- PCPs working under different employment arrangements—PCPs on full salary, PCPs with a portion of their salary at risk based on practice performance, PCPs working part-time versus full-time, PCPs in larger versus smaller group practices
- PCPs from different training origins—U.S. medical graduates and International Medical Graduates

Table 2 Study Participants

Pseudonym	Specialty	Description of participant
Wilma	Family Practice	Early career
Patrick	Internal Medicine	Later career, educational leader
Stan	Internal Medicine	Residency director
Larry	Internal Medicine	Later career, medical director
Rose	Internal Medicine	Later career
Lou	Med/Ped	Early career
Don	Family Medicine	Midcareer, IMG
Charlie	Family Medicine	Later career, former business owner
Mick	Family Medicine	Midcareer
Sam	Family Medicine	Midcareer
Tom	Med/Ped	Early career
Martin	Family Medicine	Midcareer, business owner
Francis	Family Medicine	Midcareer, former business owner
Manuel	Pediatrics	Midcareer, former academic doctor
Carol	Family Medicine	Early career, part-time, new mom
Harry	Internal Medicine	Early career
Greg	Med/Ped	Midcareer, former academic doctor
Steven	Pediatrics	Midcareer, former business owner
Peggy	Pediatrics	Later career, former owner, IMG
Paula	Internal Medicine	First-year resident
Gabrielle	Internal Medicine	Third-year resident
Linda	Internal Medicine	Later career, business owner
Monty	Internal Medicine	Third-year resident, IMG
Billy	Internal Medicine	Midcareer, business owner
Caitlyn	Internal Medicine	Early career, new mom, IMG
Rick	Internal Medicine	Later career, former business owner
Theresa	Family Medicine	Midcareer
Brad	Internal Medicine	Later career, IMG, former owner
Mark	Internal Medicine	Later career, former business owner
Sal	Internal Medicine	Midcareer, business owner
Frank	Internal Medicine	Later career, former business owner
Brian	Family Medicine	Later career, academic physician
Gary	Internal Medicine	Early career
Irene	Internal Medicine	Second-year resident, IMG
Susie	Internal Medicine	Third-year resident

(*Continued*)

Table 2   **Continued**

Peter	Pediatrics	Midcareer, former academic physician
Pam	Internal Medicine	Third-year resident
Loretta	Family Medicine	Midcareer, former business owner
Barry	Internal Medicine	Later career, former business owner
Wanda	Pediatrics	Midcareer
Jane	Family Medicine	Midcareer
Quentin	Family Medicine	Later career
Tony	Internal Medicine	Later career
Paul	Family Medicine	Early career, part-time academic
Colin	Family Medicine	Later career, former academic, IMG
Hannah	Family Medicine	Early career
Sarah	Internal Medicine	Early career, part-time, new mom
Sol	Family Medicine	First-year resident, IMG
Susan	Family Medicine	Second-year resident, IMG
Matt	Family Medicine	Later career, academic
Sally	Family Medicine	Second-year resident, IMG
Kristin	Family Medicine	First-year resident, IMG
Drew	Family Medicine	Later career, academic
Ann	Family Medicine	First-year resident, IMG
Ben	Medical student	First year
Lincoln	Family Medicine	Third-year resident, IMG
Brianna	Family Medicine	Third-year resident, IMG
Henry	Family Medicine	First-year resident, IMG
Tammy	Family Medicine	Third-year resident, IMG
Jenny	Family Medicine	Second-year resident, IMG
Camille	Family Medicine	Midcareer, academic
Donna	Family Medicine	First-year resident
Daniel	Medical student	Third year
Molly	Medical student	Second year
Zack	Medical student	Second year
Lance	Medical student	Second year
Lorenzo	Medical student	Second year
Kris	Pediatrics	Early career, part-time, new mom
Leann	Pediatrics	Midcareer, former business owner
Maura	Pediatrics	Later career
Dillon	Pediatrics	Later career
Bart	Family Medicine	Professional association leader

(*Continued*)

Table 2 **Continued**

Liz	Nonphysician	Professional association leader
Garrett	Nonphysician	Professional association leader
Bob	Internal Medicine	Professional association leader
Rhonda	Med/Ped	Third-year resident
Donald	Nonphysician	Medical reform leader
Ralph	Internal Medicine	Medical Director
Trevor	Family Medicine	Medical home leader
Shane	Internal Medicine	Midcareer
Al	Internal Medicine	Midcareer, Medical Director
Blythe	Pediatrics	Midcareer, academic
Skip	Family Medicine	Later career, Administrator
Brooke	Medical student	Third year
Louise	Medical student	Third year
Trish	Medical student	Fourth year
Blaine	Family Medicine	Third-year resident
Margo	Family Medicine	Third-year resident
Toby	Family Medicine	Second-year resident
Stephanie	Family Medicine	First-year resident

- PCPs from different racial and ethnic backgrounds
- Medical students and residents considering a primary care career and those not
- Full-time practicing PCPs and PCPs in educational or management roles
- PCPs working in different geographic locales—urban, rural, suburban

Selecting different groups of PCPs for interviews allowed a comparative approach to be used in the study. Doing comparisons when interpreting qualitative data has two advantages that strengthen study objectivity and belief in the findings: it clarifies the dominant themes, patterns, and categories of meaning that are contained in the entire data set by first revealing similarities and differences across subgroups; and it forces the validation of findings from one subgroup against those in others, leading either to more expansive explanations and descriptions of reality or specific differences in the way subgroups think and act.

Key informants working in the field of primary care were consulted early in the study for their opinions about the demographic variables selected for the PCP subgroups. These informants consisted of a high-level medical education administrator, the medical director of a large primary care network, a physician working in a managed health care insurance plan, two chairpersons of primary care academic departments, and two practicing PCPs. Several of the demographic criteria listed above are proxies for transformations now occurring within primary care, such as the greater influx of women and IMGs into primary care specialties. Other criteria sought to ensure that different groups of key stakeholders in primary care could weigh in on primary care work and changes occurring to that work, for example, PCPs across different career stages or employed in different settings.

The vast majority of study participants lived and worked in the Capital Region of New York State. This should not pose an issue in terms of representativeness since there is no valid reason to think that this geographic region differs in significant ways from others relative to the types of PCPs who work there, the kind of primary care work performed, or the types of patients encountered. The PCPs participating in the study had been raised and trained in different parts of the United States and abroad. Although limited to a single geographic area, PCPs were distributed across all of the different dimensions of the criteria noted above, so that some PCPs in the study were urban located, some were rural, some were suburban, and so on.

Almost everyone approached for an interview agreed to participate; less than a handful of the original sample could not. This is significant in the sense that practically everyone participating saw value in the study and wanted to contribute. All participation was voluntary. No incentives, financial or otherwise, were used as inducement for participation. Most of the PCPs used time during their workday to be interviewed, either very early in the morning, very late in the day, on their lunch hours, or occasionally during normal patient visit hours. Interviews lasted on average approximately sixty to seventy-five minutes. Nine of the ninety-five interviews were done by phone. The rest were performed in person with the PCP. Pseudonyms were used in the book for all physicians.

Having studied doctors and worked with them for many years, I was fortunate to have such a willing sample of whom to ask questions. It also made it relatively easy and efficient to gain detailed descriptions of everyday primary care work and career life, since PCPs wanted to talk about their experiences. Everyone participating knew the strain their field was under. It was no secret to them why someone might want to do a book about primary care work, nor why they would be asked about their work and careers in some depth. Engaged participants yield more accurate and thoughtful insights. It is not a bad thing to have people ready to tell you the truth from their own perspective, as long as there is a systematic way of parsing that truth. I was lucky to do a study of workers who were somewhat aware of their own predicaments. In my opinion, this has improved the overall accuracy of the insights gleaned for this book.

Data Collection and Analysis

A standardized interview protocol guided each interview. This was a third quality-control mechanism for enhancing study results. The protocol contained several open-ended categories of interest, such as getting PCPs to describe their typical workday, asking generally about their career experiences, finding out their likes and dislikes in relation to the changes occurring around them, and tapping into the values and beliefs that informed their lives as workers. A series of questions and probes guided the discussion within each category. Thus, for example, as PCPs described their typical workday, I was ready with additional questions that sought information on how the present workday differed from past workdays, which parts of the day PCPs felt most and least enthusiastic about, and specific ways in which PCPs managed their job duties to remain satisfied and provide good care. The interview questions remained the same across PCPs, although as the study went on patterns emerging in the data began to narrow the interview focus.

For specific PCP subgroups, questions were asked that related more to that particular group's career and work experiences. For example, it was appropriate to ask international medical graduates (IMGs) to describe their experiences as IMGs, the challenges they face in primary care that might be unique, and whether or not they have career or work approaches different from other PCP groups. Similarly with female PCPs, asking them to describe and reflect on their career experiences as women was important because it enabled differences due to gender to be identified and analyzed in detail.

One of the dangers qualitative researchers face involves the threat of the researcher "going native." This refers to a phenomenon, originating out of anthropological studies, in which researchers living among groups of people for long periods of time may get co-opted in a manner that renders their analyses biased. Because of the close and extended proximity, researchers come to identify with their subjects, see things similarly, and lose their ability to remain impartial observers. The risk of this happening with physicians as a study group, however, remains small.

Physicians, because of their lofty occupational stature, are difficult to empathize or identify with as a group, and this is probably true of many high-status professionals. Regardless of their circumstances, primary care physicians get paid well by normal standards, still have large amounts of discretion in their work, and have advantages in their jobs that other workers only dream about. My research approach was always to try and understand these types of privileged, highly skilled workers and their experiences as an outsider, as someone who could not do what they do. I believe that seeing physicians first

as a group that should be different and then letting the research process identify convergence or divergence points with other worker experiences and adaptations produces reliable sociological insights.

An additional safeguard against the problem of overidentifying with the
study group is to approach each interview in a systematic, standardized way, at
least initially, by the types of questions asked. This was done through the use
of the protocol noted above. Finally, this risk is much less when the data collection involves interviews rather than direct, extended observation with the
same group of individuals over time. Interviews yield richly detailed data in
their own right but are not as intimate as observing others do their work or live
their career.

Conducting ninety-five hour-long interviews generates a lot of data. The
interviews were digitally tape recorded. I listened to each one several times
over the study period, then used a content-analytic approach to data analysis.
This process involved listening to each interview once in its entirety, usually
within a few days of the interview itself, identifying preliminary themes, categories, or patterns of interest, defining these phenomena in terms of what they
spoke to or implied (for example, how actual work was done, how a group of
PCPs adapted to a particular reality in their workday), and then filtering the
parsed interpretations into brief descriptive vignettes that helped provide
insight into one or more aspects of the primary care workday or career experience. As the study progressed, I modified and discarded vignettes as new data
were collected and analyzed. This process produced a core set of themes, categories, and data patterns that are discussed in the previous chapters.

In order for a piece of description, larger theme, or analytic category to
assume centrality as a meaningful finding, and thus worthy of inclusion in the
overall narrative, it needed support by at least a majority of the overall PCP
sample or a particular subsample (for example, the cohort of young physicians)
to which it most referred or was applicable. Thus, for example, the chapter on
the typical PCP workday includes descriptions that more than half of the eighty-
eight PCPs interviewed (excluding the two nonphysician primary care leaders)
either supplied directly or supported when asked about it. In most cases, the
findings that made it into this book were those that were validated by the large
majority of the appropriate interview sample. Quotations from individual
respondents are used as the raw material through which these findings are
conveyed. But the quotations are illustrative of perspectives, experiences,
behaviors, and values held by significant portions of the interview sample.

There are also descriptive or analytic findings in the book that, because of
their novel or exploratory character, are based on support that falls short of the

majority rule-of-thumb. These findings were included in the overall narrative because they raise interesting questions or insights to consider around the current and future state of PCPs and primary care medicine. For example, the discussion of how electronic health records (EHR) may for some physicians change how they communicate with one another or produce unanticipated inaccuracies in patient data were not cited by a majority of PCPs. However, as there is published research supporting these insights already, explaining the idiosyncratic beliefs and experiences of a group of PCPs provides further support for how the social-psychological dynamics associated with physicians' use of technology shapes EHR implementation.

The final two chapters of the book consist of analysis that draws upon the totality of the study findings. It is within these chapters where the descriptive intent gives way to a larger set of policy and management considerations for fixing primary care. A significant contribution of the book is in presenting data that informs the prospects for effective implementation of the medical home model, looked upon with great hope by PCPs, legislators, and supporters of generalist medicine. In addition, the study results support the use of several incremental strategies to help reinvigorate the primary care physician workforce, as well as make generalist medicine more economically and socially relevant. If there is one message that the book conveys, it is that there is no single solution to the problems primary care faces today.

The study is not meant as a dry academic treatise. I have tried to present the description and supporting analysis in an accessible way. As a result, the book can be read on several levels and by different audiences. Readers may take away different conclusions or thoughts after finishing it. This is one of the rewards of qualitative research. That while a story and its underlying explanatory elements are derived systematically, people can and do see different things in the data, form their own opinions about it, and decide what it means when considering action. Each chapter provides enough detail to provoke ideas and hint at deeper questions about the state of generalist medicine and doctors today. My approach is not to try and convince the reader to adopt any particular future view of primary care. But there certainly are more believable versions of the present and future health care options, allowing individuals to engage in their own guided speculation.

Notes

Chapter 1. The Transformation of Primary Care in the United States

1. National Center for Health Statistics, "Prevalence of Overweight and Obesity among Adults, United States: 2003–2004." Available online: http://www.cdc.gov/nchs/products/pubs/pubd/hestats/overweight/overwght_adult_03.htm.
2. National Center for Health Statistics, "Prevalence of Overweight among Children and Adolescents, United States: 2003–2004." Available online: http://www.cdc.gov/nchs/products/pubs/pubd/hestats/overweight/overwght_child_03.htm.
3. American Heart Association, "Cardiovascular Disease Statistics." Available online: http://www.americanheart.org/presenter.jhtml?identifier=4478.
4. Centers for Disease Control and Prevention, "National Ambulatory Medical Care Survey: 2004 Summary." Available online: http://www.cdc.gov/nchs/data/ad/ad374.pdf.
5. American Heart Association, "Heart Disease and Stroke Statistics—2006 Update." Available online: http://circ.ahajournals.org/cgi/content/short/113/6/e85#SEC4.
6. National Diabetes Information Clearinghouse, "National Diabetes Statistics." Available online: http://diabetes.niddk.nih.gov/dm/pubs/statistics/.
7. Ibid.
8. American Diabetes Association, "Economic Costs of Diabetes in the U.S.," *Diabetes Care* 31, no. 3 (2008): 596–615.
9. Ibid.
10. Ibid.
11. Ibid.
12. National Institute of Mental Health, "Statistics." Available online: http://www.nimh.nih.gov/healthinformation/statisticsmenu.cfm.
13. Ibid.
14. Ibid.
15. National Center for Health Statistics, "Life Expectancy." Available online: http://www.cdc.gov/nchs/fastats/lifexpec.htm.
16. Centers for Disease Control and Prevention, "Trends in Aging—United States and Worldwide," *MMWR Morbidity and Mortality Weekly Report* 52, no. 6 (2003): 101–104, 106.
17. Ibid.
18. Centers for Disease Control and Prevention, "National Ambulatory Medical Care Survey: 2004 Summary." Available online: http://www.cdc.gov/nchs/data/ad/ad374.pdf.
19. K. S. Yarnall, K. I. Pollak, T. Ostbye, et al., "Primary Care: Is There Enough Time for Prevention?" *American Journal of Public Health* 93, no. 4 (2003): 635–641.
20. Patient-Centered Primary Care Collaborative, "Joint Principles of the Patient-Centered Medical Home." Available online: http://www.pcpcc.net/content/joint-principles-patient-centered-medical-home.
21. J. S. Millis, *The Graduate Education of Physicians: Report of the Citizens' Commission on Graduate Medical Education* (Chicago: American Medical Association, 1966).

22. Institute of Medicine, *Primary Care: America's Health in a New Era* (Washington, DC: National Academies Press, 1996), 27–28.

23. Ibid.

24. Kevin Goodman, "Imagining Doctors: Medical Students and the TV Medical Drama," *Virtual Mentor* 9, no. 3 (March 2007): 182–187.

25. J. Kruse, "Saving Medicare: "It's the Workforce, Stupid!" *Annals of Family Medicine* 4, no. 3 (2006): 274–275; American Academy of Family Physicians, "Facts about Family Medicine." Available online: http://www.aafp.org/online/en/home/aboutus/specialty/facts.html.

26. American Academy of Family Physicians, "Comparison of Primary Care Positions Filled with U.S. Seniors, 1996–2007." Available online: http://www.aafp.org/match2007/graph5.pdf.

27. K. E. Hauer, S. J. Durning, W. N. Kernan, et al., "Factors Associated with Medical Students' Career Choices Regarding Internal Medicine," *Journal of the American Medical Association* 300, no. 10 (2008): 1154–1164.

28. S. E. Brotherton, P. H. Rockey, and S. I. Etzel, "U.S. Graduate Medical Education, 2004–2005: Trends in Primary Care Specialties," *Journal of the American Medical Association* 294, no. 9 (2005): 1075–1082.

29. National Resident Matching Program, "Advanced Data Tables for 2007 Main Residency Match." Available online: http://www.nrmp.org/advancedata2007.pdf.

30. General Accounting Office, *Physician Workforce: Physician Supply Increased in Metropolitan and Nonmetropolitan Areas but Geographic Disparities Persisted* (Washington, DC: Government Printing Office, 2003).

31. Health Resources and Services Administration, "Physician Supply and Demand: Projections to 2020." Available online: http://bhpr.hrsa.gov/healthworkforce/reports/physiciansupplydemand/assessingadequacyofsupply.htm.

32. National Center for Health Statistics, "Ambulatory Medical Care Utilization Estimates for 2004." Available online: http://www.cdc.gov/nchs/products/pubs/pubd/hestats/estimates2004/estimates04.htm.

33. Ibid.

34. Massachusetts Medical Society, "Physician Workforce Study." Available online: http://www.massmed.org/Content/NavigationMenu/NewsandPublications/ResearchReportsStudies/PhysicianWorkforceStudy/2007MMSWorkforceStudy_full.pdf.

35. American Medical Association, *Physician Characteristics and Distribution* (Chicago: American Medical Association, 2005).

36. Cejka Search, "2006 AGMA Physician Compensation Survey." Available online: http://www.cejkasearch.com/compensation/amga_physician_compensation_survey.htm.

37. J. J. Stoddard, S. E. Brotherton, and S. F. Tang, "General Pediatricians, Pediatric Subspecialists, and Pediatric Primary Care," *Archives of Pediatrics and Adolescent Medicine* 152, no. 8 (1998): 772.

38. R. A. Garibaldi, C. Popkave, and W. Bylsma, "Career Plans for Trainees in Internal Medicine Residency Programs," *Academic Medicine* 80, no. 5 (2005): 507–512.

39. Ibid.

40. Brotherton, "U.S. Graduate Medical Education, 2004–2005: Trends in Primary Care Specialties."

41. National Resident Matching Program, "Advanced Data Tables for 2007 Main Residency Match" (see note 29).

42. American Academy of Family Physicians, "Comparison of Primary Care Positions Filled with U.S. Seniors, 1996–2007."

43. Ibid.

44. The National Residency Matching Program is an annual event in which medical school seniors select several residency programs in which they are willing to serve, and then get picked by those programs or not, depending on the students' qualifications and overall competition for the program. In this sense, students hopefully get "matched" with residency programs of their choice.

45. National Resident Matching Program, "Advanced Data Tables for 2007 Main Residency Match" (see note 29).

46. Brotherton, "U.S. Graduate Medical Education, 2004–2005: Trends in Primary Care Specialties."

47. H. C. Sox, Jr., "Quality of Patient Care by Nurse Practitioners and Physician's Assistants: A Ten-Year Perspective," *Annals of Internal Medicine* 91, no. 3 (1979): 459–468; S. Horrocks, E. Anderson, and C. Salisbury, "Systematic Review of Whether Nurse Practitioners Working in Primary Care Can Provide Equivalent Care to Doctors," *British Medical Journal* 324, no. 7341 (2002): 819–823; P. A. Ohman-Strickland, A. J. Orzano, S. V. Hudson, et al., "Quality of Diabetes Care in Family Medicine Practices: Influence of Nurse-Practitioners and Physician's Assistants," *Annals of Family Medicine* 6, no. 1 (2008): 14–22.

48. M. Laurant, D. Reeves, R. Hermens, et al., "Substitution of Doctors by Nurses in Primary Care," *Cochrane Database of Systematic Reviews* no. 2 (2005): CD001271; M. O. Mundinger, R. L. Kane, E. R. Lenz, et al., "Primary Care Outcomes in Patients Treated by Nurse Practitioners or Physicians: A Randomized Trial," *Journal of the American Medical Association* 283, no. 1 (2000): 59–68.

49. "Treatment and Cost at Minute Clinic," Available online: http://www.minuteclinic.com/en/USA/Treatment-and-Cost.aspx.

50. M. K. Scott, "Health Care in the Express Lane: Retail Clinics Go Mainstream," California HealthCare Foundation, September 2007. Available online: http://www.chcf.org/documents/policy/HealthCareInTheExpressLaneRetailClinics2007.pdf.

51. Deloitte Center for Health Solutions, "Retail Clinics: Facts, Trends and Implications" (2008). Available online: http://www.deloitte.com/dtt/cda/doc/content/us_chs_RetailClinics_230708%281%29.pdf.

52. A. Mehrotra, M. C. Wang, J. R. Lave, et al., "Retail Clinics, Primary Care Physicians, and Emergency Departments: A Comparison of Patients' Visits," *Health Affairs (Millwood)* 27, no. 5 (2008): 1272–1282.

53. Deloitte Center for Health Solutions. "Retail Clinics: Facts, Trends, and Implications."

54. Ibid.

55. E. Hing, D. K. Cherry, and D. A. Woodwell, "National Ambulatory Medical Care Survey: 2004 Summary," *Advance Data from Vital and Health Statistics*, no. 374 (2006): 1–33.

56. G. T. McMahon, "Coming to America—International Medical Graduates in the United States," *New England Journal of Medicine* 350, no. 24 (2004): 2435–2437.

57. Mary C. Noonan, Mary E. Corcoran, and Paul N. Courant, "Pay Differences among the Highly Trained: Cohort Differences in the Sex Gap in Lawyer's Earnings," *Social Forces* 84, no. 2 (2005): 853–872; Matt Huffman, "Gender Inequality across Local Wage Hierarchies," *Work and Occupations* 31, no. 3 (2004): 323–344; P. Uhlenberg and T. M. Cooney, "Male and Female Physicians: Family and Career Comparisons," *Social Science and Medicine* 30, no. 3 (1990): 373–378.

58. A. E. Wallace and W. B. Weeks, "Differences in Income between Male and Female Primary Care Physicians," *Journal of the American Medical Women's Association* 57, no. 4 (2002): 180–184; H. T. Tu and A. S. O'Malley, "Exodus of Male Physicians from Primary Care Drives Shift to Specialty Practice," *Tracking Report*, no. 17 (2007): 1–6. Available online: http://www.hschange.org/CONTENT/934/.

59. T. J. Hoff, "Doing the Same and Earning Less: Male and Female Physicians in a New Medical Specialty," *Inquiry* 41, no. 3 (2004): 301–315.

60. National Resident Matching Program, "Advanced Data Tables for 2007 Main Residency Match" (see note 29).

Chapter 2. A Typical Workday in Primary Care

1. D. K. Cherry, E. Hing, D. A. Woodwell, and E. A. Rechtsteiner, "National Ambulatory Medical Care Survey: 2006 Summary," *National Health Statistics Report*, no. 3 (2008): 1–39.

2. E. R. Dorsey, D. Jarjoura, and G. W. Rutecki, "Influence of Controllable Lifestyle on Recent Trends in Specialty Choice by U.S. Medical Students," *Journal of the American Medical Association* 290, no. 9 (2003): 1173–1178.

3. American Medical Group Association, "2008 Physician Compensation Survey." Available online: http://www.cejkasearch.com/compensation/amga_physician_compensation_survey.htm.

4. Center for Studying Health System Change, "Losing Ground: Physician Income, 1995–2003." Available online: http://www.hschange.com/CONTENT/851/.

5. Center for Studying Health System Change, "Issue Brief, January 2007: Physician Financial Incentives: Use of Quality Incentives Inches Up, but Productivity Still Dominates." Available online: http://www.hschange.com/CONTENT/905/.

6. Ibid.

7. Hemoglobin A1c involves a blood test that indicates the average amount of sugar in the blood over the prior few months. It is an important and regular part of diabetes management.

8. E. Hing, D. K. Cherry, and D. A. Woodwell, "National Ambulatory Medical Care Survey: 2004 Summary." (See note 55, chapter 1.)

9. K. G. Shojania, B. W. Duncan, K. M. McDonald, et al., "Making Health Care Safer: A Critical Analysis of Patient Safety Practices," *Evidence Report Technology Assessment (Summary)*, no. 43 (2001): i–x, 1–668; K. Grumbach and T. Bodenheimer, "Can Health Care Teams Improve Primary Care Practice?" *Journal of the American Medical Association* 291, no. 10 (2004): 1246–1251.

10. Patient-Centered Primary Care Collaborative, "Joint Principles of the Patient-Centered Medical Home." (See note 20, chapter 1.)

Chapter 3. How the Primary Care Workday Has Changed

1. Partnership to Fight Chronic Disease, "Almanac of Chronic Disease." Available online: http://www.fightchronicdisease.org/resources/almanac.cfm.

2. Kaiser Family Foundation, "Characteristics of the Medicare Population, 2006." Available online: http://facts.kff.org/chart.aspx?ch=377.

3. T. Bodenheimer, "Primary Care—Will It Survive?" *New England Journal of Medicine* 355, no. 9 (2006): 861–864.

4. J. S. Burgers, R. P. Grol, J. O. Zaat, et al., "Characteristics of Effective Clinical Guidelines for General Practice," *British Journal of General Practice* 53, no. 486 (2003): 15–19; D. A. Christakis and F. P. Rivara, "Pediatricians' Awareness of and Attitudes about Four Clinical Practice Guidelines," *Pediatrics* 101, no. 5 (1998): 825–830; M. Wolff,

D. J. Bower, A. M. Marbella, and J. E. Casanova, "U.S. Family Physicians' Experiences with Practice Guidelines," *Family Medicine* 30, no. 2 (1998): 117–121.

5. American Diabetes Association, *2007 Standards for Diabetes Care* (2008). Available online: http://care.diabetesjournals.org/cgi/reprint/31/Supplement_1/S5.

6. Institute of Medicine, *Rewarding Provider Performance* (Washington, DC.: National Academy Press, 2006); K. Grumbach, D. Osmond, K. Vranizan, D. Jaffe, and A. B. Bindman, "Primary Care Physicians' Experience of Financial Incentives in Managed-Care Systems," *New England Journal of Medicine* 339, no. 21 (1998): 1516–1521.

7. R. M. Werner and D. A. Asch, "The Unintended Consequences of Publicly Reporting Quality Information," *Journal of the American Medical Association* 293, no. 10 (2005): 1239–1244; E. C. Schneider and A. M. Epstein, "Influence of Cardiac-Surgery Performance Reports on Referral Practices and Access to Care: A Survey of Cardiovascular Specialists," *New England Journal of Medicine* 335, no. 4 (1996): 251–256; Grumbach et al., "Primary Care Physicians' Experience of Financial Incentives in Managed-Care Systems."(See note 6.)

8. Merritt, Hawkins and Associates, "2007 Survey of Primary Care Physicians." Available online: http://www.merritthawkins.com/pdf/2007_survey_primarycare.pdf.

9. Pew Internet and American Life Project, "Health Information Online." Available online: http://www.pewinternet.org/pdfs/PIP_Healthtopics_May05.pdf.

10. Pew Internet and American Life Project, "Internet Health Resources." Available online: http://www.pewinternet.org/pdfs/PIP_Health_Report_July_2003.pdf.

11. Ibid.

12. Ibid.

13. R. H. Miller and I. D. Sim, "Physicians' Use of Electronic Medical Records: Barriers and Solutions," *Health Affairs* 23, no. 2 (2004): 116–126; R. Koppel, J. P. Metlay, A. Cohen, et al., "Role of Computerized Physician Order Entry Systems in Facilitating Medication Errors," *Journal of the American Medical Association* 293, no. 10 (2005): 1197–1203; C. M. DesRoches, E. G. Campbell, S. R. Rao, et al., "Electronic Health Records in Ambulatory Care—a National Survey of Physicians," *New England Journal of Medicine* 359, no. 1 (2008): 50–60.

Chapter 4. Leaving Hospital Work Behind

1. C. J. DeFrances and M. J. Hall, "2005 National Hospital Discharge Survey," *Advanced Data*, no. 385 (2007): 1–19.

2. A. D. Auerbach, E. A. Nelson, P. K. Lindenauer, et al., "Physician Attitudes toward and Prevalence of the Hospitalist Model of Care: Results of a National Survey," *American Journal of Medicine* 109, no. 8 (2000): 648–653.

3. R. M. Wachter and L. Goldman, "The Hospitalist Movement 5 Years Later," *Journal of the American Medical Association* 287, no. 4 (2002): 487–494.

4. Ibid.

5. J. Coffman and T. G. Rundall, "The Impact of Hospitalists on the Cost and Quality of Inpatient Care in the United States: A Research Synthesis," *Medical Care Research and Review* 62, no. 4 (2005): 379–406.

6. P. K. Lindenauer, M. B. Rothberg, P. S. Pekow, et al., "Outcomes of Care by Hospitalists, General Internists, and Family Physicians," *New England Journal of Medicine* 357, no. 25 (2007): 2589–2600.

7. Institute of Medicine, *To Err is Human* (Washington, DC: National Academy of Sciences, 1999).

8. Wachter and Goldman, "The Hospitalist Movement 5 Years Later." (See note 3.)

Chapter 5. The Routine and Nonroutine of Primary Care Work

1. E. Hing, D. K. Cherry, and D. A. Woodwell, "National Ambulatory Medical Care Survey: 2003 Summary," *Advanced Data from Vital and Health Statistics* 365 (2005): 1–48.
2. Ibid.
3. Ibid.
4. Hing, Cherry, and Woodwell, "National Ambulatory Medical Care Survey: 2004 Summary." (See note 55, chapter 1.)
5. M. Bazargan, R. W. Lindstrom, A. Dakak, et al., "Impact of Desire to Work in Underserved Communities on Selection of Specialty among Fourth-Year Medical Students," *Journal of the National Medical Association* 98, no. 9 (2006): 1460–1465; Garibaldi, Popkave, and Bylsma, "Career Plans for Trainees in Internal Medicine Residency Programs." (See note 38, chapter 1.)
6. A "procedure" in primary care may be thought of in terms of hands-on treatment by PCPs for patients including, but not limited to, casting and splinting for broken or sprained bones, needle aspirations of cysts, debridement and stitching of wounds, screening procedures such as flexible sigmoidoscopies of the colon, and EKGs and stress tests.
7. One of the true benefits of using clinical practice guidelines is to reduce disparities in how different patient populations are diagnosed and treated. By asking physicians in a given specialty such as primary care to conform to the same basic processes and outcomes of care for all their patients, the risk of introducing bias or subjectivity into the clinical decision making process is reduced greatly.
8. C. B. Forrest and R. J. Reid, "Prevalence of Health Problems and Primary Care Physicians' Specialty Referral Decisions," *Journal of Family Practice* 50, no. 5 (2001): 427–432.
9. Lexipro is a commonly used drug used to treat major depressive disorder and generalized anxiety disorder.
10. W. O. Cooper, P. G. Arbogast, H. Ding, et al., "Trends in Prescribing of Antipsychotic Medications for U.S. Children," *Ambulatory Pediatrics* 6, no. 2 (2006): 79–83.
11. Ibid.
12. National Center for Health Statistics, "National Survey of Child Health." Available online: http://www.cdc.gov/nchs/about/major/slaits/nsch.htm.
13. Ibid.
14. Ibid.
15. National Institute of Mental Health, "Statistics." (See note 12, chapter 1.)
16. Ibid.
17. National Mental Health Association, "America's Mental Health Survey 2001." Available online: http://www1.nmha.org/pdfdocs/mentalhealthreport2001.pdf.
18. R. Paulose-Ram, M. A. Safran, B. S. Jonas, et al., "Trends in Psychotropic Medication Use among U.S. Adults," *Pharmacoepidemiology and Drug Safety* 16, no. 5 (2007): 560–570.

Chapter 6. Younger and Older Physicians in Primary Care

1. E. R. Dorsey, D. Jarjoura, and G. W. Rutecki, "Influence of Controllable Lifestyle on Recent Trends in Specialty Choice by U.S. Medical Students," *Journal of the American Medical Association* 290, no. 9 (2003): 1173–1178.
2. Ibid.; Garibaldi, Popkave, and Bylsma, "Career Plans for Trainees in Internal Medicine Residency Programs" (see note 38, chapter 1); G. Xu, S. L. Rattner, J. J. Veloski, et al., "A National Study of the Factors Influencing Men and Women Physicians' Choices

of Primary Care Specialties," *Academic Medicine* 70, no. 5 (1995): 398–404; R. A. Rosenblatt and C. H. Andrilla, "The Impact of U.S. Medical Students' Debt on Their Choice of Primary Care Careers: An Analysis of Data from the 2002 Medical School Graduation Questionnaire," *Academic Medicine* 80, no. 9 (2005): 815–819.

3. Cejka Search and American Medical Group Association, "2007 Physician Retention Survey, Supplemental Edition." Available online: http://www.cejkasearch.com/pdf/2007-Physician-Retention-Survey-SE_web.pdf; Merritt, Hawkins and Associates, "2007 Survey of Primary Care Physicians." Available online: http://www.merritthawkins.com/pdf/2007_survey_primarycare.pdf.

4. Massachusetts Medical Society, "Physician Workforce Study." (See note 34, chapter 1.)

5. Ibid.

6. Cejka Search and American Medical Group Association, "2007 Physician Retention Survey, Supplemental Edition." (See note 3.)

7. Ibid.

8. N. W. Sobecks, A. C. Justice, S. Hinze, et al., "When Doctors Marry Doctors: A Survey Exploring the Professional and Family Lives of Young Physicians," *Annals of Internal Medicine* 130, no. 4, pt. 1 (1999): 312–319.

9. Merritt, Hawkins and Associates, "2008 Review of Physician and CRNA Recruitment Incentives," Available online: http://www.merritthawkins.com/pdf/mha-2008-incentive-survey.pdf.

10. Ibid.

11. Ibid.

12. Ibid.

13. Merritt, Hawkins and Associates, "Summary Report: 2006 Review of Physician Recruitment Incentives," Available online: http://www.merritthawkins.com/pdf/2006_incentive_survey.pdf.

14. Association of American Medical Colleges, "Curriculum Directory," Available online: http://services.aamc.org/currdir/about.cfm.

15. Association of American Medical Colleges, "Curriculum Directory, School Curricula," Available online: http://services.aamc.org/currdir/section2/courses.cfm.

16. C. Bianco, "How Becoming a Doctor Works," Available online: http://people.howstuffworks.com/becoming-a-doctor9.htm.

17. S. E.Weinberger, L. G. Smith, and V. U. Collier, "Redesigning Training for Internal Medicine," *Annals of Internal Medicine* 144, no. 12 (2006): 927–932; K. M. Ludmerer and M. M. Johns, "Reforming Graduate Medical Education," *Journal of the American Medical Association* 294, no. 9 (2005): 1083–1087.

18. P. Starr, *The Social Transformation of American Medicine* (New York: Basic Books, 1982).

19. Cejka Search and American Medical Group Association, "2007 Physician Retention Survey, Supplemental Edition." (See note 3.)

20. Ibid.

21. Ibid.

22. Ibid.

Chapter 7. Women in Primary Care

1. "MomMD: Connecting Women in Medicine." Available online: http://www.mommd.com/.

2. D. L. Roter, J. A. Hall, and Y. Aoki, "Physician Gender Effects in Medical Communication: A Meta-Analytic Review," *Journal of the American Medical Association* 288, no. 6 (2002): 756–764.

3. J. A. Hall, "Do Patients Talk Differently to Male and Female Physicians? A Meta-Analytic Review," *Patient Education and Counseling* 48, no. 3 (2002): 217–224.

4. Association of American Medical Colleges, "Table 2: Women Medical School Applicants," Available online: www.ama-assn.org/ama/pub/category/12913.htm.

5. S. E. Brotherton and S. I. Ethel, "Graduate Medical School Education, 2005–2006," *Journal of the American Medical Association* 296, no. 9 (2006): 1154–1169.

6. Ibid.

7. American Medical Association, *Physician Characteristics and Distribution in the U.S., 2008 Edition* (Chicago: American Medical Association, 2008).

8. G. Xu, S. L. Rattner, J. J. Veloski, et al., "A National Study of the Factors Influencing Men and Women Physicians' Choices of Primary Care Specialties," *Academic Medicine* 70, no. 5 (1995): 398–404.

9. M. C. Harris, J. Marx, P. R. Gallagher, and S. Ludwig, "General vs. Subspecialty Pediatrics: Factors Leading to Residents' Career Decisions over a 12-Year Period," *Archives of Pediatric and Adolescent Medicine* 159, no. 3 (2005): 212–216.

10. H. T. Tu and A. S. O'Malley, "Exodus of Male Physicians from Primary Care Drives Shift to Specialty Practice." (See note 58, chapter 1.)

11. S. G. Gabbe, M. A. Morgan, M. L. Power, et al., "Duty Hours and Pregnancy Outcome among Residents in Obstetrics and Gynecology," *Obstetrics and Gynecology* 102, no. 5, pt. 1 (2003): 948–951; J. L. Klevan, J. C. Weiss, and S. M. Dabrow, "Pregnancy during Pediatric Residency: Attitudes and Complications," *American Journal of Diseases in Children* 144, no. 7 (1990): 767–769.

12. Cejka Search and American Medical Group Association, "2007 Physician Retention Survey, Supplemental Edition." (See note 3, chapter 6.)

13. D. L. Roter, J. A. Hall, and Y. Aoki, "Physician Gender Effects in Medical Communication: A Meta-Analytic Review," *Journal of the American Medical Association* 288, no. 6 (2002): 756–764.

14. Ibid., 756

15. Hall, "Do Patients Talk Differently to Male and Female Physicians? A Meta-Analytic Review." (See note 3.)

16. Mara S. Aruguete and Carlos A. Roberts, "Gender, Affiliation, and Control in Physician-Patient Encounters," *Sex Roles: A Journal of Research* 42, no. 1/2 (2000): 107–118.

17. Roter, Hall, and Aoki, "Physician Gender Effects in Medical Communication: A Meta-Analytic Review." (See note 13.)

18. Ibid.

19. J. W. Kenagy, D. M. Berwick, and M. F. Shore, "Service Quality in Health Care," *Journal of the American Medical Association* 281, no. 7 (1999): 661–665.

20. W. Levinson, D. L. Roter, J. P. Mullooly, et al., "Physician-Patient Communication: The Relationship with Malpractice Claims among Primary Care Physicians and Surgeons," *Journal of the American Medical Association* 277, no. 7 (1997): 553–559; R. Tamblyn, M. Abrahamowicz, D. Dauphinee, et al., "Physician Scores on a National Clinical Skills Examination as Predictors of Complaints to Medical Regulatory Authorities," *Journal of the American Medical Association* 298, no. 9 (2007): 993–1001.

21. M. C. Fang, E. P. McCarthy, and D. E. Singer, "Are Patients More Likely to See Physicians of the Same Sex? Recent National Trends in Primary Care Medicine," *American Journal of Medicine* 117, no. 8 (2004): 575–581.

22. Alice H. Eagly and Blair T. Johnson, "Gender and Leadership Style: A Meta-Analysis," *Psychological Bulletin* 108, no. 2 (1990): 233–256.

23. A. E. Wallace and W. B. Weeks, "Differences in Income between Male and Female Primary Care Physicians," *Journal of the American Medical Women's Association* 57, no. 4 (2002): 180–184.

24. Roter, Hall, and Aoki, "Physician Gender Effects in Medical Communication: A Meta-Analytic Review" (see note 13); D. Mechanic, D. D. McAlpine, and M. Rosenthal, "Are Patients' Office Visits with Physicians Getting Shorter?" *New England Journal of Medicine* 344, no. 3 (2001): 198–204.

Chapter 8. International Medical Graduates in Primary Care

1. American Medical Association, "IMGs in the United States," Available online: http://www.ama-assn.org/ama/pub/category/211.html.

2. Ibid.

3. J. K. Iglehart, "The Quandary over Graduates of Foreign Medical Schools in the United States," *New England Journal of Medicine* 334, no. 25 (1996): 1679–1683.

4. American Medical Association, "International Medical Graduates: A Discussion Paper" Available online: http://www.ama-assn.org/ama1/pub/upload/mm/18/img-workforce-paper.pdf.

5. American Medical Association, "IMGs in the United States." (See note 1.)

6. G. P. Whelan, N. E. Gary, J. Kostis, et al., "The Changing Pool of International Medical Graduates Seeking Certification Training in U.S. Graduate Medical Education Programs," *Journal of the American Medical Association* 288, no. 9 (2002): 1079–1084.

7. J. R. Boulet, D. B. Swanson, R. A. Cooper, et al., "A Comparison of the Characteristics and Examination Performances of U.S. And Non-U.S. Citizen International Medical Graduates Who Sought Educational Commission for Foreign Medical Graduates Certification: 1995–2004," *Academic Medicine* 81, no. 10, Suppl. (2006): S116–119.

8. J. J. Norcini, J. R. Boulet, G. P. Whelan, et al., "Specialty Board Certification among U.S. Citizen and Non-U.S. Citizen Graduates of International Medical Schools," *Academic Medicine* 80, no. 10, Suppl. (2005): S42–45.

9. S. S. Mick and M. E. Comfort, "The Quality of Care of International Medical Graduates: How Does It Compare to That of U.S. Medical Graduates?" *Medical Care Research and Review* 54, no. 4 (1997): 379–413.

10. S. Y. Lee, William Dow, Virginia Wang, et al., "Use of Deceptive Tactics in Physician Practices: Are There Differences between International and U.S. Medical Graduates?" *Health Policy* 67 (2004): 257–264.

11. Ibid.; H. C. Kales, A. R. DiNardo, F. C. Blow, et al., "International Medical Graduates and the Diagnosis and Treatment of Late-Life Depression," *Academic Medicine* 81, no. 2 (2006): 171–175.

12. B. Starfield and G. E. Fryer, Jr., "The Primary Care Physician Workforce: Ethical and Policy Implications," *Annals of Family Medicine* 5, no. 6 (2007): 486–491.

13. A Foley catheter consists of a tube placed in the bladder to allow continuous urine drainage.

14. American Medical Association, "IMGs in the United States." (See note 1.)

15. World Health Organization, "World Health Report 2000," Available online: http://www.who.int/whr/2000/en/index.html.

16. Brotherton, Rockey, and Etzel, "U.S. Graduate Medical Education, 2004–2005: Trends in Primary Care Specialties." (See note 28, chapter 1.)

17. Ibid.

18. P. A. Pugno, A. L. McGaha, G. T. Schmittling, et al., "Results of the 2007 National Resident Matching Program: Family Medicine," *Family Medicine* 39, no. 8 (2007): 562–571.

19. M. E. Whitcomb and R. S. Miller, "Participation of International Medical Graduates in Graduate Medical Education and Hospital Care for the Poor," *Journal of the American Medical Association* 274, no. 9 (1995): 696–699.

20. D. C. Goodman, "The Pediatrician Workforce: Current Status and Future Prospects," *Pediatrics* 116, no. 1 (2005): e156–173; S. S. Mick and S. Y. Lee, "International and U.S. Medical Graduates in U.S. Cities," *Journal of Urban Health* 76, no. 4 (1999): 481–496; A. Hagopian, M. J. Thompson, E. Kaltenbach, and L. G. Hart, "Health Departments' Use of International Medical Graduates in Physician Shortage Areas," *Health Affairs* (Millwood) 22, no. 5 (2003): 241–249.

21. D. L. Howard, C. D. Bunch, W. O. Mundia, et al., "Comparing United States versus International Medical School Graduate Physicians Who Serve African-American and White Elderly," *Health Services Research* 41, no. 6 (2006): 2155–2181.

22. D. Polsky, P. R. Kletke, G. D. Wozniak, and J. J. Escarce, "Initial Practice Locations of International Medical Graduates," *Health Services Research* 37, no. 4 (2002): 907–928.

23. American Medical Association, "International Medical Graduates: A Discussion Paper." (See note 4.)

24. G. T. McMahon, "Coming to America—International Medical Graduates in the United States," *New England Journal of Medicine* 350, no. 24 (2004): 2435–2437.

25. Howard, Bunch, Mundia, et al., "Comparing United States versus International Medical School Graduate Physicians Who Serve African-American and White Elderly." (See note 21.)

26. McMahon, "Coming to America—International Medical Graduates in the United States." (See note 24.)

27. Ibid.

Chapter 9. The Medical Home: Primary Care Savior?

1. Patient-Centered Primary Care Collaborative, "Joint Principles of the Patient-Centered Medical Home." (See note 20, chapter 1.)

2. Institute of Medicine, *To Err Is Human*. (See note 7, chapter 4.)

3. Ross Koppel, J. P. Metlay, A. Cohen, et al., "Role of Computerized Physician Order Entry Systems" (see note 13, chapter 3); D. Pittet, A. Simon, S. Hugonnet, et al., "Hand Hygiene among Physicians: Performance, Beliefs, and Perceptions," *Annals of Internal Medicine* 141 (2004): 1–8; Institute of Medicine, *Preventing Medication Errors* (Washington, DC: National Academy of Sciences, 2004).

4. Institute for Healthcare Improvement, "The Chronic Care Model." Available online: http://www.ihi.org/IHI/Topics/ChronicConditions/AllConditions/Changes/.

5. TransforMED, "Commonwealth Fund Teams with America's Family Physicians," Available online: http://www.transformed.com/news-eventsdetailpage.cfm?listingID =10.

6. The "RBRVS" stands for "resource-based relative value scale" and was a payment system implemented in the early 1990s that was supposed to address the disparities in reimbursement between primary and specialty care when identical services are provided, by making reimbursement more uniform across specialties through factoring in the amount of resources and time spent by any physician performing the service or procedure. The RBRVS replaced the "usual and customary" fee approach

used, which favored nonprimary care specialists who traditionally billed more for their work and received greater payments even when doing the same work as a primary care physician.

7. Roter, Hall, and Aoki, "Physician Gender Effects in Medical Communication: A Meta-Analytic Review." (See note 13, chapter 7.)

Chapter 10. No Quick Fix: An Incremental Approach to Helping Primary Care

1. Massachusetts Medical Society, "Physician Workforce Study." (See note 34, chapter 1.)
2. Deloitte Center for Health Solutions. "Retail Clinics: Facts, Trends, and Implications." (See note 51, chapter 1.)
3. Merritt Hawkins and Associates, "Review of Physician and CRNA Recruiting Incentives" (2008). Available online: www.merritthawkins.com.
4. Ibid.
5. General Accounting Office, *Physician Workforce: Physician Supply Increased in Metropolitan and Nonmetropolitan Areas but Geographic Disparities Persist* (see note 30, chapter 1); Bureau of Labor Statistics, "Physician Assistants," in *Occupational Outlook Handbook* 2008–2009. Available online: http://www.bls.gov/oco/ocos081.htm.
6. Deloitte Center for Health Solutions. "Retail Clinics: Facts, Trends, and Implications." (See note 51, chapter 1.)
7. S. D. Block, N. Clark-Chiarelli, A. S. Peters, and J. D. Singer, "Academia's Chilly Climate for Primary Care," *Journal of the American Medical Association* 276, no. 9 (1996): 677–682; S. Schafer, W. Shore, L. French, et al., "Rejecting Family Practice: Why Medical Students Switch to Other Specialties," *Family Medicine* 32, no. 5 (2000): 320–325.
8. Block, Clark-Chiarelli, Peters, and Singer, "Academia's Chilly Climate for Primary Care" (See note 7.)
9. Ibid.
10. Ibid.
11. C. J. Bland, L. N. Meurer, and G. Maldonado, "Determinants of Primary Care Specialty Choice: A Non-Statistical Meta-Analysis of the Literature," *Academic Medicine* 70, no. 7 (1995): 620–641.
12. Ibid.
13. Schafer, Shore, French, et al., "Rejecting Family Practice: Why Medical Students Switch to Other Specialties" (see note 7); M. D. Schwartz, W. T. Basco, Jr., M. R. Grey, et al., "Rekindling Student Interest in Generalist Careers," *Annals of Internal Medicine* 142, no. 8 (2005): 715–724; C. J. Martini, J. J. Veloski, B. Barzansky, et al., "Medical School and Student Characteristics That Influence Choosing a Generalist Career," *Journal of the American Medical Association* 272, no. 9 (1994): 661–668; E. H. Osborn, "Factors Influencing Students' Choices of Primary Care or Other Specialties," *Academic Medicine* 68, no. 7 (1993): 572–574.
14. Ibid.
15. Bland, Meurer, and Maldonado, "Determinants of Primary Care Specialty Choice: A Non-Statistical Meta-Analysis of the Literature." (See note 11.)
16. A. Kalet, M. D. Schwartz, L. J. Capponi, et al., "Ambulatory versus Inpatient Rotations in Teaching Third-Year Students Internal Medicine," *Journal of General Internal Medicine* 13, no. 5 (1998): 327–330; Garibaldi, Popkave, and Bylsma, "Career Plans for Trainees in Internal Medicine Residency Programs" (see note 38,

chapter 1); W. J. Kassler, S. A. Wartman, and R. A. Silliman, "Why Medical Students Choose Primary Care Careers," *Academic Medicine* 66, no. 1 (1991): 41–43.

17. R. M. Fincher, "The Road Less Traveled—Attracting Students to Primary Care," *New England Journal of Medicine* 351, no. 7 (2004): 630–632; M. E. Whitcomb and J. J. Cohen, "The Future of Primary Care Medicine," *New England Journal of Medicine* 351, no. 7 (2004): 710–712.

18. Dorsey, Jarjoura, and Rutecki. "Influence of Controllable Lifestyle on Recent Trends in Specialty Choice by U.S. Medical Students." (See note 1, chapter 6.)

19. Hauer, Durning, Kernan, et al., "Factors Associated with Medical Students' Career Choices Regarding Internal Medicine." (See note 27, chapter 1.)

20. U.S. Department of Health and Human Services, "Reimbursement of Mental Health Services in Primary Care Settings," Available online: http://download.ncadi.samhsa .gov/ken/pdf/SMA08–4324/SMA08–4324.pdf.

21. H. Leigh, D. Stewart, and R. Mallios, "Mental Health and Psychiatry Training in Primary Care Residency Programs. Part II. What Skills and Diagnoses Are Taught, How Adequate, and What Affects Training Directors' Satisfaction?" *General Hospital Psychiatry* 28, no. 3 (2006): 195–204; E. R. Park, T. J. Wolfe, M. Gokhale, et al., "Perceived Preparedness to Provide Preventive Counseling: Reports of Graduating Primary Care Residents at Academic Health Centers," *Journal of General Internal Medicine* 20, no. 5 (2005): 386–391; H. Leigh, D. Stewart, and R. Mallios, "Mental Health and Psychiatry Training in Primary Care Residency Programs. Part I. Who Teaches, Where, When and How Satisfied?" *General Hospital Psychiatry* 28, no. 3 (2006): 189–194.

22. H. P. Chin, G. Guillermo, S. Prakken, and S. Eisendrath, "Psychiatric Training in Primary Care Medicine Residency Programs: A National Survey," *Psychosomatics* 41, no. 5 (2000): 412–417.

23. Wachter and Goldman, "The Hospitalist Movement 5 Years Later." (See note 3, chapter 4.)

24. S. Z. Pantilat, P. K. Lindenauer, P. P. Katz, and R. M. Wachter, "Primary Care Physician Attitudes Regarding Communication with Hospitalists," *American Journal of Medicine* 111, no. 9B (2001): 15S–20S.

25. S. A. Schroeder and R. Schapiro, "The Hospitalist: New Boon for Internal Medicine or Retreat from Primary Care?" *Annals of Internal Medicine* 130, no. 4, pt. 2 (1999): 382–387.

Appendix: How the Study Was Conducted

1. A. Strauss, *Qualitative Analysis for Social Scientists* (New York: Cambridge University Press, 1987).

Index

About the Author

Timothy Hoff is an associate professor of Health Policy and Management at the University at Albany School of Public Health, where he codirects the Policy and Management Track of the Master's in Public Health Program. He is a two-time recipient of the school's excellence in teaching award. He has published over thirty-five lead-authored articles, and his research has won national awards from the American Sociological Association, Academy of Management, and Society for Applied Anthropology. He has served in a variety of prominent service roles, including chair of the Health Care Management Division of the Academy of Management, editorial board member for the health services journals *Medical Care Research and Review* and *Health Care Management Review*, and member of the health services research study section of the Agency for Healthcare Research and Quality. In 2008, he was appointed by the Institute of Medicine as a member of the Committee on Review of Priorities in the National Vaccine Plan. Before coming to academia, Dr. Hoff worked for a decade as an administrator and consultant in the health care industry. His areas of expertise are primary care, health care workforce issues, patient safety, and health care quality.

Available titles in the Critical Issues in Health and Medicine series: